Hair Loss Prevention

THROUGH NATURAL REMEDIES

*A Prescription
for
Healthier Hair*

Ken Peters • David Stuss • Nick Waddell

Apple Publishing Company Ltd.
220 East 59th Avenue
Vancouver, British Columbia
Canada v5x 1x9
Tel (604) 325.2888 • Fax (604) 322.6978

ISBN: 0-9695272-6-8

For Tim

Contents

Introduction

AMERICAN MEDICAL ASSOCIATION figures show that forty per cent of all men will experience some degree of hair loss by the time they're forty. The number rises to sixty five per cent by the time they reach seventy. The figures are alarmingly high for women, as well.

These numbers sound familiar, even acceptable to our ears. Yet simple cross cultural and historical comparison reveals that few societies rival ours when it comes to the attention given to hair loss.

It is, at first glance, a seemingly trivial cosmetic change. Some men even feel they look better without hair. For most others, however, it is important. Important enough to sustain the four billion dollar industry that hair loss is here in North America.

If, in terms of physical health, hair loss were an isolated phenomenon concerning only the health of follicles and scalp, it would likely still be a four billion dollar industry. The condition is infrequently linked to general health in our society. Perhaps we have made an unconscious assumption that nothing can be done. If so, this is unfortunate, for perspective and examination consistently point to hair loss as symptomatic of larger, broader based lifestyle related problems. Diet is the most dramatic and influential of these, and, as such, is our primary focus.

For comparison's sake we will detail a few conventional treatments for hair loss.

One of the more popular procedures is the hair transplant. During a hair transplant small pieces of skin containing tufts of hair are removed from the back and sides of the head. These 'plugs' are then surgically inserted into the thinning areas at a cost of thousands of dollars, depending on how many plugs must be inserted. Unfortunately, the quality of the finished product can vary greatly; much depends upon the skill of the surgeon. In order for the job to appear natural the surgeon must possess both good surgical technique and artistic ability.

Another specialized surgical procedure known as scalp reduction has been used with some success. In a series of operations the scalp is cut and a section of flesh is shifted forward to cover balding areas. The patient must wear a dressing until the scalp heals and then, usually about six weeks later, the operation is repeated. The process often takes more than a year to complete.

A new technique currently popular is the hair weave, which is the least invasive (i.e. non-surgical) of the cosmetic cover-ups. Here real hair of the same color is woven into one's hair base until the balding area is hidden. It will last for months through regular activities and then must be upgraded. Some patients find the weave to be irritating and unnatural.

The only product sanctioned by the USFDA and Health and Welfare Canada as a hair loss treatment is Minoxidil. Originally created as a high blood pressure medication by Upjohn Pharmaceuticals, researchers observed that it caused patients to sprout hair all over their bodies. Originally produced in tablet form the medicine was reformulated into a lotion called Rogaine, which received FDA approval in 1988. In July, 1989, the FDA banned all non-prescription creams and lotions which claimed to cure or prevent baldness. Because Rogaine, even applied topically, still has the potential to alter a user's blood pressure it is available only with a doctor's prescription. Rogaine is designed to be applied to the scalp twice a day at a cost of at least sixty dollars per month. In order for the product to be effective one must continue to use the product forever, or the resulting new growth will eventually fall out. Dr. Shapiro, a dermatologist specializing in hair loss research and treatment at the University of British Columbia's Adult Hair Clinic claims that about thirty per cent of users will grow new hair, but only eight per cent of that hair is 'cosmetically acceptable.' Even if one ignores the cost and associative difficulties of using Rogaine the risk of side effects is considerable. Upjohn itself has warned of possible negative side effects including 'increased heart rate, rapid weight gain or edema, difficulty in breathing, worsening of or new onset of angina pectoris.' Many other potential side effects are mentioned, which, along with those mentioned above, have been reported in the users of the tablet form prescribed to lower blood pressure. Even though the dosage is much lower in the topical solution it will still enter the bloodstream via the skin of the scalp.

The remedies in this book, gathered around the world from the pages of tradition, history, and science share the distinction of being free of negative side effects. In fact, many of them offer positive health benefits. Some of these products, such as Polysorbate 80 and Biotin have shown to be effective at halting, even reversing hair loss in scientific double blind studies. Still, manufacturers of these products may make no legal claims as to their effectiveness. This situation exists because the law requires that in order to claim that a product will 'cure' an ailment one must first obtain FDA (in Canada Health and Welfare) approval. Obtaining such approval is a lengthy, expensive, and somewhat political proposition, requiring extensive scientific experimentation and study. The cost of such a procedure is often hundreds of thousands of dollars. This kind of investment is only warranted when a company can obtain an exclusive patent on a given product. This can guarantee a return on investment and a profit level worthy of the financial risk involved. No one can control the rights to common substances such as vitamins (biotin), food emulsifiers (polysorbate 80), and herbs. Only drugs fall into this category.

The bottom line is this: if you are already bald there is very little you can do to reverse it naturally. This book will best benefit those with thinning hair, or those interested in prevention. However, all who use the techniques and methods included will follow a safe path towards improving general health and longevity.

CHAPTER ONE

Your Hair

THE SCALP IS A COMPLEX ORGAN containing between 100,000 and 150,000 hair follicles, an equal number of pigment and sebaceous glands, and thousands of sweat glands. There are at least half a million glands in the scalp that serve the purpose of growing hair, and to function properly they must be well nourished. Starve these glands and hair loss begins.

The development of hair starts when epidermal cells form a follicle; a hollow, cylindrical depression in the skin or scalp. Follicles produce Keratin, a protein comprised of carbon, hydrogen, nitrogen, sulfur and oxygen, which forms ninety seven per cent of the hair shaft. The rest of the shaft is moisture. Hair, especially if brittle or thin, is sensitive enough to act as a natural barometer. In humid conditions it can absorb up to forty per cent of its' own weight in water.

Hair development goes through three stages: anagen, the growing stage, catagen, the transitional stage, and telogen, the resting stage. At any given time approximately eighty-five per cent of the hair is in the growing stage, fifteen per cent is in the resting stage. Each individual hair may grow for two to six years, then the follicle goes into a resting phase for about three months, during which there is no growth. When the hair follicle begins production again it starts to grow a new hair shaft which pushes the old one out. Normally one loses fifty to a hundred hairs per day, and ideally gains the same number of new ones.

Sebaceous glands within follicles lubricate the scalp and hair with an oily, rich, yellowish substance called sebum. With its' ability to absorb and retain large amounts of moisture, the sebum also fills skin tissue, keeping it plump and firm. A deficiency of sebum leads to a dry scalp that becomes dry and scaly; without it hair becomes brittle, and may break or split. An excess of sebum has also been linked to hair loss (See "EFAs") The sebaceous glands require essential fatty acids in combination with a variety of minerals to produce sebum.

Once hair is visible it is literally dead tissue (much like fingernails). Hence, it is unable to repair itself, leaving it vulnerable to permanent damage. The only growing or live portion of the hair is its' root

Cross Section of the Scalp

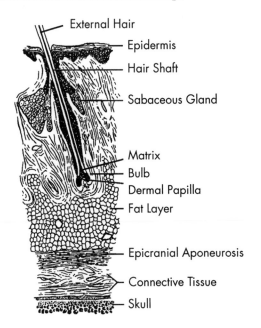

External Hair
Epidermis
Hair Shaft
Sabaceous Gland
Matrix
Bulb
Dermal Papilla
Fat Layer
Epicranial Aponeurosis
Connective Tissue
Skull

which is located at the base of the follicle. The root envelops a tiny bulb shaped organ called the papilla (the hair bud) which is filled with capillaries that deliver nutrients to the hair. The papilla are present at birth. Each grows a couple of hairs. When you lose one that hair is gone forever, much like a tooth. Both Iron and Iodine help the glands provide nourish-ment to the papilla.

The hair shaft consists of three layers: the medulla (inner layer), the cortex (middle layer), and the cuticle (outer covering). The medulla is the core of the shaft. As well as absorbing beneficial substances it serves as the supporting structure for the strand of hair. The cortex, protected by the cuticle, consists of rope-like protein fibers and hair color pigments. If the cuticle is damaged the cortex is exposed, allowing for moisture loss. The cortex then unravels in split ends and mid-shaft damage which can lead to breakage. The cuticle is made of hard, transparent cells that overlap each other like the scales of a fish. These cells, called imbrications, are hinged to open and close.

When these overlapping cells lie flat the hair feels smooth and looks shiny. Since it is the cuticle which gives elasticity and resiliency to the hair its condition largely determines the hair's appearance. Hair growth in humans averages about one one-hundredth of an inch per day, and according to the scientific community does not grow faster when it is cut. However, hair length may influence the rate of growth, slowing down once the length exceeds ten inches. Hair grows fastest in the summer and slowest in the winter. Growth speeds up under heat and friction (massage), but slows down when exposed to long periods of cold. The structure and strength of a gray hair is no different from that of a colored hair, and while the beginning of graying often corresponds with the start of hair loss there is no evidence linking the two.

Causes of Hair Loss

THINNING HAIR, a withering of the hair in its' follicle, can begin at any age after puberty. It can precede actual baldness (in which the follicle atrophies and stops producing hair altogether) by ten years or more. Alopecia (the medical term for baldness or hair loss) is believed to be hereditary and generally incurable. The idea that nutritional deficiencies and inherited eating patterns actually create this condition has received very little research or support in the west. The fact that, for example, blond haired men are more predisposed to baldness than dark haired men, or Caucasians more than Blacks or Asians is often attributed to genetic factors. However, investigation on the subject suggests that environment may play a greater role than previously suspected.

What is commonly referred to as Male Pattern Baldness was recognized as far back as the time of Hippocrates. He observed that castrated males never go bald. Further on, it was discovered that balding men who were castrated as a result of wounds received during World War Two often regained their hair. More recently, studies have shown that such males, who no longer produce significant levels of testosterone, will sometimes lose their hair after being injected with androgens. Interestingly, as soon as the injections were stopped, the patients regained their hair.

To understand how Male Pattern Baldness works it is first important to become familiar with the hormones involved. There are two types of sex hormones: estrogen, produced primarily in the ovaries, and androgens, the male specific hormones produced mostly in the testicles, predominantly in the form of testosterone. Testosterone is of special importance. Certain hair follicle cells are genetically predetermined to accept testosterone, while others are not. A limited amount of both types of hormone is also produced by the adrenal glands. It is this additional hormonal activity of the adrenals that can trigger hair loss.

Male Pattern Baldness is seen as operating on a biological clock. It is understood that hair follicles have a growing and resting cycle. When testosterone enters the follicles of those genetically predisposed to MPB, the hair follicles noticeably increase their production of the enzyme testosterone 5-alpha reductase. In turn, this enzyme converts testosterone to a hormone called dihydrotestosterone (DHT). Follicles exposed to DHT enter the resting phase and begin to atrophy and shrink. At the same time the galea aponeurotica membrane in the scalp becomes thickened and inelastic, cutting off circulation. Eventually the follicle structure becomes so withered and shallow the scalp can no longer sustain hair growth. The hair growth cycle is altered and follicles begin to spend more time in the resting phase, and less in the growing phase. Hair continues to fall out at the normal rate, but it is not replaced. Eventually there are no macroscopic hairs left in the area. (The atrophied follicles are not necessarily dead, however, and may be induced to resume growth with proper stimulation.)

The adrenal hormones protect the body in stressful situations through the 'fight or flight' response. Adrenaline is released into the bloodstream, increasing heart rate, blood pressure and energy levels. In this heightened state the body is better able to deal with threatening situations. However, the body is unable to distinguish between these acute threats and the long-term stresses associated with modern life. Over time, this raises blood pressure and blood fat levels, increasing the risk of heart attack or stroke. Muscles and bones are weakened and the immune system is impaired.

Overstimulated adrenal glands also produce extra androgens, thereby raising testosterone levels.

Steroid hormones such as testosterone are made from cholesterol, a substance naturally present in the body. When steroid hormones are needed, additional cholesterol is drawn from the circulation, converted to the hormone, and quickly reintroduced to the bloodstream. A high intake of animal foods, notably dairy products, eggs and fatty meats, brings an excess of cholesterol into the body. The mechanism of constantly stressed adrenal glands combined with excess cholesterol can lead to the high level of androgens that is associated with Male Pattern Baldness.

After menopause many women will experience symptoms of hair loss, as well as an increased amount of facial hair. When a woman enters into menopause, or loses her period due to a high level of physical activity or dieting, her estrogen levels drop. Estrogen binds

Cross Section of the Hair Follicle

The three stages of development of the Hair Follicle are:

A) **Anagen** (growth)   B) **Catagen** (transition)   C) **Telogen** (rest).

The follicle stops producing a hair at the Telogen stage.

At this point, it shrivels up, and the bulb largely degenerates.

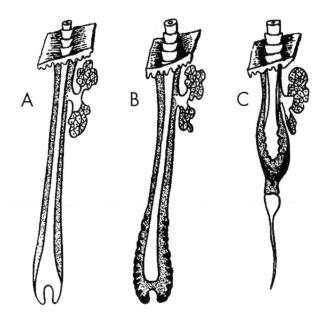

excess testosterone to proteins called globulins and lowers the free-form testosterone levels in the blood. Lowered levels of estrogen thus allow free testosterone levels to rise, leading to hair loss by the same mechanism as Male Pattern Baldness. The fine vellus hairs of the body, which are colourless and soft, are also converted into terminal hairs, which are coarser and pigmented.

A withdrawal from birth control pills, as well as childbirth, will cause a fall in estrogen levels. Hair loss after childbirth will return to normal levels after a few months. When the ovaries reduce their production of estrogen, as well as the related female hormone progesterone, the body is usually able to compensate by producing the required hormones through the adrenal glands. However, when the body is overstressed and the adrenal glands are exhausted this backup system is insufficient. In this way the connection between the adrenal system and hair loss is as significant for women as it is for men. It is interesting to note that the conventional problems associated with menopause in the western world are uncommon in Japan. Because, until recently, red meat (which raises testosterone levels) was rarely consumed by the Japanese, and soy foods (which contain estrogen like substances) were widely consumed the women of Japan were able to maintain high enough estrogen levels after menopause to avert menopausal problems.

The Prostate and Male Pattern Baldness

THE PROSTATE is a cluster of small, doughnut shaped sex glands. They encircle the urethra (the tube which conveys urine and semen) just below the bladder. Though all the functions of the prostate are not yet clear, its' most direct purpose is to contract during ejaculation. It squeezes the seminal fluid into and through the urethral tract. Because the prostate is located so close to the urethra, any problem with the prostate can hinder the free flow of urine.

It is interesting to note that as little as a hundred years ago prostate problems were rarely mentioned in medical literature. This implies a link to a modern lifestyle (i.e. diet). Indeed, the connection between prostate cancer and a diet high in animal fats has been clearly established. About fifty per cent of men between the ages of forty and sixty have the most common disorder of the prostate gland: benign prostatic hyperplasia (BPH). Symptoms of BPH include increased frequency of urination, waking at night to empty the bladder, and reduced force and caliber of urination.

BPH is believed to be caused by an accumulation of testosterone in the prostate. Within the prostate the enzyme known as 5-alpha reductase converts the male sex hormone, testosterone, into another more potent hormone known as dihydrotestosterone (DHT), the same hormone linked to Male Pattern Baldness. DHT controls the division of cells in the prostate. This compound stimulates the prostate cells to multiply excessively, eventually causing the prostate to enlarge.

Normally DHT would be excreted from the prostate gland in sufficient quantity to prevent enlargement. However, if there is an imbalance between the male hormones (androgens) then the DHT is not adequately excreted, causing the prostate to swell. Examination of an enlarged prostate usually reveals three to four times the normal levels of DHT.

The greatest danger that follows Benign Prostatic Hyperplasia is that of a possible malignant change occurring. The metabolites (breakdown products) of cholesterol are cancer producing , and have a tendency to accumulate in the prostate gland. These metabolites initiate a degeneration in the prostate cells which can promote prostatic enlargement. There is a high correlation between prostate cancer and fat consumption. Worldwide autopsies reveal that wherever the diet is similar to a typical North American one (i.e. high animal fat consumption) nearly twenty-five per cent of all men develop latent cancer of the prostate by the time they reach old age. The Journal of the National Cancer Institute recently reported that men who ate red meat at least five times a week had a two and a half times greater risk of developing prostate cancer than did men who ate red meat less than once a week (based on a study of 51,000 men). Countries with the highest prostate cancer death rates are Denmark, The Netherlands, US, Canada, and the UK. Those with the lowest include: The Philippines, El Salvador, Japan, Colombia, and Mexico.

Diets high in saturated fat and cholesterol have a tendency to clog up the arteries. This reduces and sometimes obstructs blood flow to the heart and brain, not to mention the scalp. A thereosclerosis also tends to reduce blood flow to all the organs, including the reproductive ones, often producing impotence in older men. A study by the Chief of Urology at Metropolitan Hospital in New York found that men with DHT had 80% more cholesterol in their blood than those without the condition.

Maintaining cholesterol levels at a safe limit involves watching fat consumption. But it also must include restricting sugar intake and ensuring an adequate amount of fiber. Both sugar and fiber are involved in the body's ability to process and utilize cholesterol. Another good reason to include a high fiber content in your diet is the need for bowel regularity. Constipation is a frequent symptom accompanying BPH. It is quite possible that the long term increase in pressure creates congestion in the lower pelvic region, where the prostate lies.

The mineral zinc has been shown to inhibit the activity of 5-alpha reductase, the enzyme which aids in the conversion of testosterone to DHT. Unfortunately, the Zinc levels in the average man are seldom adequate (See "Minerals"), and with this deficiency comes higher 5-alpha reductase levels. The prostate gland normally contains about ten times more zinc than any other organ in the body. As a preventative supplement fifteen to thirty mg per day is usually sufficient. If one already has an enlarged prostate more research is advised, for this requires a complete supplementation program in conjunction with dietary controls. There are indications that those with BPH also have an imbalance in the quantities of and ratios between their essential fatty acids Men that showed a high plasma level of alpha linoleic acid had eight times the risk of developing prostate cancer than a control group. The Townsend Letter for Doctors reported a limited, uncontrolled study in which BPH patients were supplemented with EFAs. "All nineteen subjects... showed a diminution of residual urine, with twelve of nineteen having no residual urine by the end of several weeks of treatment."

A soon to be familiar face in the war against hair loss shows up in the European research into prostate problems. Nettle Root Extract has been used successfully to exert a decongestive action on the prostate, thus relieving the discomfort resulting from enlargement of this gland. Nettles are rich in vitamins, minerals, and lipids. They have been shown to actually inhibit the activity of 5-alpha reductase, as well as supporting endocrine gland activity.

Perhaps more substantial than Nettles in the treatment of BPH is the use of Saw-Palmetto Berries. A standardized, fat soluble extract of the fruit of Serenoa Repens (Saw Palmetto Berries) can alleviate the major symptoms of BPH in a surprisingly effective manner. The extract is effective at preventing the conversion of testosterone to

DHT, and also inhibits DHT's binding to cellular and nuclear receptor sites, thereby increasing the breakdown and excretion of DHT. A suggested dose of Saw Palmetto is 160 mg of a standardized extract taken twice per day. Pumpkin seeds, a traditional remedy for prostate problems are not only a high source of zinc, but also contain traces of the hormones normally produced by the prostate. It too inhibits the conversion of testosterone to dihydro-testosterone. Bee pollen also features these three elements, and has been used for BPH.

Now that the mechanism of prostate disorders is understood pharmaceutical companies have begun studies of drugs known as 5-alpha reductase inhibitors, which block the action of this enzyme. One such drug, known as Proscar, is marketed by Merck and Co., of Rathway, NJ, as a treatment for non-cancerous prostate enlargement. Saw-Palmetto extract is not only significantly less expensive than Proscar, but has shown a thirty per cent higher success rate in reducing symptoms. Already research has begun with Proscar to determine whether it will be a 'new Minoxidil,' so to speak. Though it doesn't produce the feminizing characteristics of other anti-androgen medications the results so far have been 'disappointing.'

Dietary Concerns

WHILE IT IS TRUE that hair is essentially dead tissue, hair growth at the root level is a living part of your body. As such, it is as dependent on the nutritional quality of your blood as any other part of your body. If the diet does not contain all the necessary vitamins, minerals, proteins, essential fatty acids and trace elements, the blood will be deficient. Correspondingly, hair growth will be unhealthy and weak.

A variety of nutritional deficiencies have been associated with hair loss, especially those involving the B-complex vitamins. It is well established that severe malnutrition will cause hair loss, and while this extreme is uncommon in the western world, subclinical B-complex deficiencies are extremely common. The refining of whole grains removes a primary source of B vitamins, as does boiling or oversteaming vegetables, since the B's are water soluble. The modern diet is often lacking in raw leafy greens, another major source of many B vitamins. To make matters worse, the vitamins that are ingested are often diverted in order to facilitate the digestion of refined carbohydrates, including sugar, white flour and other refined grains whose own B vitamins have been stripped away in the refining process.

Stimulants such as alcohol, caffeine, nicotine and sugar, have a two-sided effect on the body in relation to hair loss. They rob the body of nutrients they lack as they pass through the system. They also affect the adrenal glands. Long-term use of these substances will leave the adrenal glands in a stressed and depleted state, creating additional nutritional demands on the body and, more significantly, raising androgen levels. The lost nutrients and higher levels of male hormones are both of negative consequence for healthy hair.

All steroid hormones produced in humans are made from cholesterol, a substance manufactured within the body by the liver. A high intake of animal foods (especially dairy products like butter and cheese as well as fatty meats) brings an excess of cholesterol into the system. High levels of cholesterol are associated with high levels of DHT, the byproduct of testosterone that is linked to both Male Pattern Baldness and prostate problems.

In 1955 a New York scientist, Dr. Eugene Foldes, followed up on Swedish experiments linking salt intake to hair loss. Dr. Foldes supected that salt actually accumulated in some tissues, disturbing their function. To test his theory he simply administered a diuretic to a test group. This would cause a body to excrete fluid, and with it excess salt from the tissues. The results were impressive; in some patients hair loss was reduced by as much as 60%.

Reducing the amount of salt in the tissues of the scalp is as simple as reducing salt intake. As the necessary daily requirement for sodium is only 0.2 to 0.6 grams, this is easily obtained in a normal diet without adding any salt at all. A safer alternative to common tale salt is sea salt. which contains a healthier balance of minerals. Should you wish to experiment with a diuretic, it is strongly recommended that you purchase a herbal diuretic from a health food store, which is a safe and effective alternative to diuretic drugs and their inherent dangers.

When a diet is low in fibre, undigested food remains in the system longer than is necessary. This causes bacterial changes (fermentation) which not only inhibit the quantity and quality of nutrients entering the bloodstream but also allow for the entry of more toxic byproducts. Since the hair follicles are dependent on the quality of nutrients they receive from the blood, a low fiber diet will also affect hair growth negatively.

Hair is dominantly comprised of protein, so it follows that one should be assured of an adequate daily protein intake. Protein malnutrition in the western world occurs mostly among strict vegetarians, people on crash diets and those with severely abnormal or poor eating habits. Excessive hair loss begins after two or three months as the body shifts the hair growth cycle into the resting phase in an attempt to conserve protein. Do not, however, make the mistake of eating too much protein in an attempt to prevent hair loss, as a high-protein diet is detrimental to your general health. Carl Pheiffer of the Brain-Bio Institute, in Princeton, NJ, and M.D. Michael Colgan determined that when protein exceeds 15 to 20% of the diet, the body enters a 'negative mineral balance,' resulting in hair loss akin to that caused by too little protein. Total protein intake should not exceed 30 to 40 grams a day; the daily protein requirement of a 170 lb man doing light work is 25 to 30 grams. Remember, most of the men in China, India, Japan and Mexico have handsome, thick hair throughout their lives, yet by western standards they live on a very low protein diet. Studies of the nutritional habits of the people in these countries show their diets to be rich in the nutritive elements necessary for hair growth. The Chinese eat a great variety of vegetables, which they do not overcook. Their diet is rich in rice, soybeans, and high-protein/low cholesterol seafoods. Chinese cuisine is high in the vitamins, minerals and essential fatty acids important for healthy hair. Traditional Japanese diets incorporate plenty of seafood and seaweeds rich in Iodine, one of the most important nutrients in hair health. In Mexico and India, rice and beans are a dietary staple, and the consumption of fresh whole fruits and vegetables is the norm.

Another important dietary concern is nutritional malabsorption. A nutritious diet is practically worthless if the body is unable to absorb the elements it requires. As the body ages, the production of stomach acids decreases. This weakness shows up first in the digestion of protein. The more obvious signs of poor digestion are gas, heartburn and bloating. A feeling of exhaustion following a meal could indicate that too much energy is being spent in digestion.

The digestive process involves several different stages. The first begins in the mouth, where chewing helps convert solid food to a liquid medium. Saliva initiates the digestive process, breaking down carbohydrates and preparing foods for the digestive tract. Chewing triggers the secretion of stomach acids and initiates peristalsis (the movement of food through the digestive tract). If these signals are not received a heavy burden is placed on the digestive system.

The next level of digestion occurs in the stomach. A variety of enzymes begin to break down the food. The pancreas both stores and produces these enzymes. Enzymes are stored when raw food is eaten, and are used up in the digestion of cooked food. The typical North American diet, which overemphasizes cooked and processed foods, will produce a pancreas that by middle age is unable to produce adequate amounts of enzymes. This may be treated therapeutically with a full-spectrum enzyme complex, available in health food stores. However, chronic use of such products, as well as 100% raw food diets, will weaken the pancreas by making it 'lazy' and can lead to dependence. A more permanent solution involves changing the ratio of raw to cooked foods consumed. The pancreas can also be stimulated to produce its own enzymes with herbal combinations and liquid whey products.

The third stage of digestion occurs when hydrochloric acid is secreted for further breakdown of food. Insufficient stomach acid is a common problem which can, unexpectedly, result in heartburn. The excessive use of antacids can worsen digestive disturbances in the long run. An easy way to determine whether or not an imbalance exists is to take a tablespoon of apple cider vinegar or lemon juice at the onset of heartburn. If symptoms clear up, you are deficient in stomach acids; if they are aggravated, stomach acid is excssive. Apple cider vinegar is an inexpensive and effective digestive aid for those with hydrochloric acid deficiency. Five minutes before a meal mix a third of a teaspoon with one teaspoon water, swish about in the mouth, and swallow.

After passing through the stomach food is almost entirely digested. It enters the intestines, where the 'friendly' bacteria commonly known as acidophilus become involved. Acidophilus is the dominant bacteria in a healthy gut. Its digestion-related functions include a role in enzyme production and the transportation of vitamins and minerals into the bloodstream. Other fuctions include immune system support, colon cancer prevention, control of cholesterol levels and the regulation of hormonal fluctuations. Friendly bacteria are destroyed by many facets of modern lifestyles. Among these are smoking, chlorinated tap water, rancid oils and food poisoning. Antibiotics are by far the most destructive, for they do not discriminate between the good and bad bacteria in the body. Low levels of acidophilus can lead to high levels of undesirable bacteria, often associated with numerous health problems including candida overgrowth. Without active supplementation the digestive system will never fully recover the beneficial bacteria lost.

Symptoms of a lack of friendly bacteria include gas and flatulence, bad breath, pimples and blemishes, bloating, indigestion and headaches. While most traditional diets contain a cultured food rich in friendly bacteria (eg. yogurt, sauerkraut, sourdough, miso), they serve a maintenance purpose only. These foods are not sufficient to counteract antibiotics, nor can they serve a therapeutic, restorative function. Acidophilus is best-suited to this purpose. It can be purchased in a concentrated, encapsultated form in the refridgerator section of most health food stores. It should ideally be taken on an empty stomach with water, in order to bypass harsh stomach acids so that it may implant and colonize in the intestines. Acidophilus may be taken after a meal to alleviate heartburn caused by excessive stomach acid, In this case the best form to use would be one in a calcium base.

There is a dangerous tendency in the standard American diet to create a buildup of fat and mucus deposits along the intestinal walls. This layering is the result of a high fat , high protein diet combined with low fibre levels. This condition prevents nutrients from passing through the intestinal wall into the bloodstream. Nutritional deprivation is the result, and it becomes increasingly difficult to feel satiated by a meal. The safest and easiest way to eliminate this buildup is to add a fiber agent to the diet. This will also keep cholesterol levels down and prevent congestion in the prostate area. Psyllium husks, commercially available in bulk or in the product 'Metamucil,' are especially well suited to this task. Psyllium swells with water and pushes old matter through the intestines, scraping the buildup off intestinal walls. This scraping action will also remove some friendly bacteria, so an acidophilus suppplement is recommended. Mix a level tablespoon of psyllium in six ounces of water or juice, drink, then follow with another six ounces of liquid and an acidophilus capsule. This should be done on an empty stomach, preferably early in the morning, or at least one half hour before a meal. For maintenance purposes once or twice a week is sufficient. Intestinal cleansing requires the same dosage for up to ten days.

Vitamins

IT IS, OF COURSE, NECESSARY that all nutrients be provided to the body in sufficient amounts for one to attain and maintain good health. The quality and quantity of one's hair is a reflection of that health. However, it is beyond the scope of this book to be a primer on the proper levels of all required nutrients necessary for general well being. Therefore, in this section, and the following ones on minerals and other supplements we shall focus only on those nutrients and products with a track record of being useful in maintaining healthy hair, preventing hair loss, and regenerating hair growth. The nutritional needs and tolerances of an individual will vary according to body size, metabolism and metabolic type, age, diet, genetics, etc. We advise you seek more information, either through books, a nutritional consultant, or in discussions at your local vitamin shop before deciding to take large quantities of any of the substances mentioned. While foodstuffs containing high levels of vitamins and minerals are safe to experiment with, isolated nutrients require more careful thought.

Vitamin A is basic for maintaining healthy bones, eyes, glands, hair, skin and teeth. In conjunction with silica and zinc it helps prevent drying and clogging of the sebaceous glands. A deficiency can lead to dandruff and dry, dull hair. It causes the scalp to thicken , trapping oil and perspiration beneath the surface. In order for the thyroid gland to take in enough iodine (its' major nutrient) to function properly there must be a sufficient amount of Vitamin A. Iodine is essential for healthy hair.

Vitamin A deficiency can also lead to a degeneration of the pituitary gland. The pituitary gland controls the structure and output of the thyroid gland by means of a thyroid-stimulating hormone. The thyroid hormone acts as a sort of carburetor to regulate both cell metabolism and the use of nutrients (aided by oxygen) utilized to generate heat and energy. The most common symptoms of hypothyroidism are chronic fatigue, cold hands or feet pale skin, nervousness, brittle nails and poor memory. Of particular interest are the symptoms of dry, coarse skin and hair, and hair loss. To test yourself for an under active thyroid simply keep a thermometer by your bed. In the morning place the thermometer under your arm for fifteen minutes. Keep very still, as the slightest movement can affect body temperature. A temperature of 97.6 degrees F or lower may indicate an under active thyroid.

Of the vitamin A destroyers in modern life the most dramatic are air pollution (including smoking), overly bright lighting, aspirin, barbiturates, antibiotics, laxatives, and some cholesterol lowering drugs. If you feel you are especially at risk take Vitamin A in pill form. Most adults can safely consume 10 000 iu per day as a maintenance dosage. Seek advice before taking higher doses though, as Vitamin A is a fat soluble nutrient, and as such is stored by the body, unlike water-soluble nutrients (including the B-vitamins) which wash through the body each day. In some instances a high dose of Vitamin A can produce undesirable side effects, such as dry skin and inflamed hair follicles, and so it is important to pay attention to your body while taking such a dosage. Vitamin A rich foods include: Alfalfa, apricots, beets, broccoli, cantaloupe, carrots, swiss chard, fish liver oils, animal livers, kale, parsley, red peppers, sweet potatoes, spinach, yellow squash, and watercress. Most green or yellow fruits and vegetables are high in Vitamin A.

Biotin, a member of the Vitamin B complex, has shown some success at slowing hair loss. Deficiencies in B vitamins such as Biotin are quite common, and the symptoms are wide ranging. They include: poor appetite, lack of energy, sleeplessness, dry skin, dermatitis, graying and/or falling hair, and a disturbed nervous system. Biotin is also valuable for its' high sulfur content. Sulfur is one of the main cleansing agents in our bodies, as well as an element necessary for healthy hair growth (See "Minerals")

Biotin works synergistically with vitamins B-2, B-6, B-3, and A. It serves the function of a coenzyme, assisting in cell growth, fatty acid production, the metabolization of carbohydrates, fats, and proteins, and the utilization of the B-Vitamins. Its' antagonists include egg whites, antibiotics, alcohol, sulfa drugs, and rancid fats. Standard supplemental dosages are in the range of 300 mcg, (this is micrograms, not milligrams) though some people take three times as much per day. Remember, isolated B-Vitamins require a B-Complex backup. This is required to facilitate their own absorption, and to prevent high levels of one B robbing the body of another. Some rich sources of biotin include egg yolk, brown rice, cauliflower, mushrooms, salt-water fish, soybeans, poultry, and nutritional yeast.

One exciting study done with Biotin took the approach of using it externally. In a series of tests involving balding men Biotin was used instead of estrogen (commonly used in scientific experiments to counteract testosterone, also believed to be responsible for male pattern baldness) in a penetrating cream applied to the scalp daily. The cream, with a Biotin content between .25 and 1% also contained Niacin, a histamine releasing form of vitamin B-3. The Niacin was included to stimulate cell growth and reproduction as well as to increase circulation. In addition to the cream the men used a special shampoo used to reduce hair breakage, which included the amino acids L-cysteine and L-methionine, two of the most important components in the protein that comprises hair. Unlike the estrogen cream there were absolutely no side effects to the Biotin program. Of the nearly twelve hundred men in the study (ranging in age from fifteen to sixty nine) eighty nine per cent showed a definite reduction in hair fallout over a six to eight week period. Daily hair loss fell from one hundred to three hundred and fifty hairs per day down to an average of less than fifty. Preliminary data (the study was incomplete at the time it was published) indicated that an unspecified amount of re-growth occurred in about fifty to seventy-five per cent of the subjects, with the best results occurring among the younger men involved. There is currently on the market a biotin based lotion, backed up with a shampoo and conditioner, all similar to those used in the above-mentioned study.

Inositol, another part of the Vitamin B complex is a cell membrane stabilizer and antioxidant that has a protective effect on the hair follicles, perhaps by shielding them from membrane damage caused by oxidized cholesterol in the scalp. One of the most important functions of Inositol is to combine with choline to form lecithin, which metabolizes fats and cholesterol. This not only wards off coronary disease, but by preventing the hardening and narrowing of the arteries it also helps to keep a healthy blood and nutrient flow to the scalp and hair roots. Inositiol deficiency has been shown to cause hair loss and graying, in various degrees. Other deficiency symptoms include constipation, eczema, and abnormalities of the eyes. Inositol has a somewhat sedative like effect, and so is beneficial for insomnia, and can relieve mild hypertension through gradually lowering blood pressure. Clearly, this is a supplement to be considered where stress is playing a major role in hair loss. Excessive caffeine intake will rob the body of Inositol, therefore heavy coffee and black tea drinkers should consider supplementation. Amounts recommended range from 100 mg to 200 mg per day. Inositol is found naturally in unprocessed whole grains, citrus fruits, nutritional yeasts, unrefined molasses, legumes and lecithin.

Niacin is the form of Vitamin B-3 currently often used as a cholesterol lowering agent. However, the dosages required to do this (up to 2000 mg per day) have become questionable due to the possibility of liver damage. For most purposes, including the circulatory benefits which concern us at this time, there is little or no danger, as one would only have to 'flush.' Begin with 25 mg, taken with a meal. Increase until a slight, red rash appears on the skin. A distinct tingling sensation will occur. This is caused by the release of histamine, which will flush blood to the extremes of the capillaries, to obvious circulatory benefit. Most people flush at around the level of 100 mg. One may increase the dosage gradually, if necessary. After a few days of this you will notice that the rash has taken on the appearance of an even sunburn, indicating that the once closed capillaries have opened up to receive blood flow. Should the reaction be too unpleasant, take Vitamin C or aspirin, both of which are anti-histamines. You will literally feel increased blood flow to the scalp. Choose a time to ingest the Niacin when you will be home for awhile, as your skin will remain a bright red for about twenty minutes.

Should its cholesterol lowering properties be of interest to you, then you should know that 200 mcg of Chromium along with 100 mg of Niacin has a similar effect to taking large doses of niacin alone, without the drawbacks. Recommended are yeast-extracted chromium, or the patented product 'Chromemate.' Do not confuse niacin, a vasodilator, with the other form of B-3, Niacinamide, which is used therapeutically for other purposes. Niacinamide will not cause flushing, nor histamine release, and serves no function for reversing hair loss. Aside from the wonders Niacin performs on circulation, a dominant metabolite of the histamine it releases is Heparin, perhaps the most important mucopoly-saccharide involved in hair growth. Mucopolysacharides work with Collagen as the biological cement that holds tissues together. As mentioned above, histamine release is essential for cell growth and reproduction. As it is only possible to receive the histamine releasing effects from Niacin as an oral supplement we shall dispense with mentioning those foods high in B-3.

PABA (Para-aminobenzoic acid) is another member of the B Vitamin family. Much like Inositol it is an antioxidant and a membrane stabilizer. Acting as a coenzyme, PABA participates in the breakdown and utilization of protein, and assists in the formation of red blood cells. PABA has shown some success at retarding hair loss and reversing premature graying caused by stress or nutritional deficiency.

In "Diseases of Metabolism" Dr. F.A. Evans revealed that falling hair was reported by some obese women after several months on an extremely restricted diet (350 to 450 calories per day). These were diets high in protein and not believed to be grossly deficient in any nutrients, yet the women in question lost large amounts of hair. When PABA was supplemented hair growth returned. In a related small scale study daily doses of 1000 to 3000 mg of PABA gave a response similar to that of Inositol: a reduction of hair loss, but no new growth, and in some cases a darkening of graying hair. As a part of total dietary regimen PABA is usually recommended in doses of around 100 mg per day. Sulfa drugs may rob the body of PABA. The best sources of it are mushrooms, cabbage, sunflower seeds, oats, spinach, eggs, whole grains, and nutritional yeast.

Pantothenic Acid (B-5), often referred to as the 'Anti-Stress Vitamin,' plays a key role in the production of the adrenal hormones, and is involved in the formation of antibodies. It aids in the utilization of other vitamins and helps to metabolize fats, carbohydrates, and proteins. Bulb and follicle atrophy, hair loss and graying are B-5 deficiency symptoms, as are adrenal exhaustion, hypoglycemia, fatigue, irritability, nervous system disorders, skin problems and premature aging. Pantothenic acid has been able to increase the life span of laboratory animals by over twenty per cent, and at the same time produced increased stamina and endurance. It has also proven helpful in treating anxiety and depression. Recommended dosages range from 100 mg three times a day for hair loss programs, to a total of 1000 mg per day for other disorders. The richest food source of B-5 is Royal Jelly, a product harvested from bees. This is perhaps the main reason why Royal Jelly is touted as a longevity substance and is so popular for a wide range of ailments, including fatigue. Royal Jelly also contains every essential nutrient considered necessary to support human life. Other food sources of B-5 include eggs, beans, salt-water fish, fresh vegetables, bee pollen, and L-Cysteine.

As a group, the B-Vitamins are of particular value in helping to counteract the harmful effects of high stress levels. Members of the Vitamin B-complex group that play a supportive role in hair and follicle health include B-2, B-6, and Folic Acid. The B's, however, are interdependent; they require one another for proper body assimilation. Because they never exist in isolation naturally it is best to take a B-Complex supplement, in addition to any particular ones you may wish to focus on. As with most vitamins (and minerals) high levels of B's are most effective when taken in divided doses, with food, throughout the day. Three times a day is most efficient.

Another supplement, Bee Pollen, has been mentioned in many anecdotal reports by those who had originally lost hair. After taking pollen over a long period of time (initially for another reason) a new strong growth of hair appeared. Bee Pollen contains 35% protein, half of which is in the form of free amino acids which can be immediately assimilated by the body. It is also high in Vitamins A, C, D. E, all the B's and lecithin. A complete 'super-food,' Bee Pollen contains every substance needed to maintain life. This nutritional powerhouse has been used around the world for centuries and is presently very popular with athletes. Being rich in the amino acid L-Cysteine may be one reason why Pollen has a beneficial effect on arresting hair loss and stimulating new growth. The composition of hair is approximately 8% L-Cysteine, an amino formed from L-Methionine, with an extremely high Sulphur content.

L-Cysteine is utilized as a component of some vitamin compounds on the market that are designed to aid hair growth, but it may also be purchased in its pure form. This may be worth considering since it has a wide range of other important benefits. It helps to detoxify harmful toxins, protects and preserves cells, and promotes fat burning and muscle building. As well as protecting cells from the effects of radiation, it protects the brain and liver from the damaging effects of alcohol and cigarettes.

High doses of L-Cysteine can lead to an increase in Cystine, the oxidized and unstable form of L-Cysteine, unless high doses of Vitamin C are taken. This also helps prevent the formation of Cystine kidney or bladder stones. It is recommended that three times as much Vitamin C as L-Cysteine be taken. Since the average dose taken as part of a hair-rebuilding regimen is 500 mg twice a day, make sure that you take three grams (3000 mg) of Vitamin C in divided doses each day. Some of the richer food sources of L-Cysteine are eggs, alfalfa, carrot, beet, cabbage, cauliflower, onion, garlic, kale , horseradish, brussel sprouts, legumes, apples, currants, pineapples, hazelnuts, and filberts.

Two other vitamins important to hair growth are C and E. Vitamin C has a multitude of health maintenance functions. It plays a key role in Collagen formation, improves scalp circulation, and is required for adrenal gland function, which is necessary to keep stress levels under control. Daily dosage should be in the range of 500 to 3000 mg, in a buffered (i.e. non acidic) form to avoid stomach irritation or diarrhea. A good Vitamin C product should include 'Bioflavanoids,' a co-factor of C which helps to strengthen veins and cappillaries.

Vitamin E also improves circulation to the scalp by increasing oxygen uptake. E deficiency symptoms include hair loss and brittle hair. Supplementation with E can strengthen the heart and immune system. Begin with 400 i.u per day, and work up to 800 i.u. during the course of a few weeks. Always use natural source Vitamin E (referred to on the label as 'd'alpha tocopherol') rather than the synthetic form derived from petroleum (dl'alpha tocopherol). The synthetic form is not only far less biologically available to the body, but actually blocks E-receptor sites, making it difficult for the body to assimilate E in the future. Supplementation with Vitamin E is contraindicated in cases of high blood pressure. As is the case with all isolated nutrients, if you have a serious illness you should consult your physician before beginning supplementation.

And important fact to remember about vitamins and their assimilation is that they and minerals require each other in sufficient amounts ('co-factors') in order to facilitate their respective absorption. Therefore, if one is lacking you will not properly absorb the other. The implication here is that you must have a good, well rounded diet in order to properly utilize these supplements. Just as no single food-stuff will guarantee good health, no single, isolated supplement can guarantee healthy hair.

Minerals

SOME YEARS AGO the sheep farmers of the Great Lakes regions found they were having difficulty getting their sheep to grow wool. This area, like many others, was known to have Iodine deficient soil. Therefore, the grazing plants were similarly deficient. This type of problem is quite common, and easily remedied. Once Iodine was added to the sheep's rations the quality and quantity of their wool immediately improved. Our well being could be greatly affected by such rational and direct thinking regarding diet. Certain mineral deficiencies are so common in our part of the world that the resulting conditions (thyroid problems, prostate cancer, hair loss) are taken as a matter of course. yet preventative measures can be taken quite simply, and produce remarkable results.

Your hair's roots must receive proper mineral nourishment in order to perform the function of growing and maintaining a healthy head of hair. Once denied these nutrients the scalp tissues begin to break down, and hair loss results. While all minerals are required in balanced proportions to promote good health, some of them stand out as key players in the health of your hair.

Iodine deficiency in humans first manifests itself as prematurely gray, dry and stringy hair with lackluster quality, and degrees of hair loss. By regulating the thyroid gland with adequate amounts of Iodine, allowing it to issue a steady flow of the hormone Thyroxin, the hair follicles receive the nourishment necessary for healthy growth. Thyroxin works with body proteins to metabolize and deliver nutrients to the millions of capillary blood vessels, lymph vessels, nerve endings, and sebaceous glands, nourishing and rejuvenating them. The Thyroxin penetrates into the layer of fat beneath the scalp, feeding the hair follicles and prompting the sebaceous glands to secrete sebum.

As a supplement, the Iodine found in seaweeds and ocean plants is most effective. In this form it is naturally balanced with co-factors, and is almost identical to the form found in the thyroid gland. One of the better oceanic sources of Iodine is called Irish Moss, a powerhouse of vitamins and minerals. The rich alkaline nature of Irish Moss helps to maintain the body's delicate acid–alkaline balance, an important factor in regulating the flow of thyroxin from the thyroid gland. Irish Moss also contains Vitamins A, D, E and K, as well as Calcium, Sodium, Phosphorus, Potassium, Sulfur, and Essential Fatty Acids.

Sea water Algaes, now quite common on the market in pill form, are also a good source of both Iodine and the family of nutrients that work together to form thyroxin. The seaweed Kelp is the most commonly recommended and available source of Iodine. It also contains a wide range of vitamins and other minerals, including Biotin, Inositol, PABA, Calcium, Sulfur, and Zinc. Kelp should be taken in quantities of six to ten tablets per day. This may seem like a lot to take, but remember that this is a food (a 'super food', if you will) and not a vitamin or mineral pill, which is a concentrated and isolated nutrient.

Prior to dramatically increasing your daily intake of organic Iodine with supplementation it is advisable to first discontinue the use of synthetic Iodine, which is added to all common table salt. Switching to non-iodized sea salt is a good idea. This helps curb the potential for Iodine overload. Synthetic Iodine, because it is not provided with its' natural co-factors, does not assimilate well, and many people consume too much salt to begin with. This synthetic Iodine builds up in the body, often overwhelming the thyroid and inhibiting its' proper function. Trace amounts of natural Iodine are present in sea salt. While ocean plants are our prime source of Iodine, there are other rich food sources. These include salmon, sardines, and other seafoods, lima beans, molasses, eggs, potatoes with skins, watercress, and garlic.

According to Denham Harman, MD., a professor of medicine and biochemistry at the University of Nebraska, the diets of most American men are deficient in zinc. Zinc deficiency can cause derangement of the hormonal rhythms, including that of the thyroid gland. It is essential for the proper functioning of more than seventy enzyme systems. Zinc's involvement in hair health stems from its role in protein synthesis, collagen formation, and the maintenance of a healthy immune system. Its dosage in supplemental form ranges from fifteen to fifty mg per day. But caution must be used in self-prescribing zinc. While an insufficient amount will impair the immune system, so will an excess. Zinc can also rob the body of Copper, one of its co-factors. One interesting thing to note about Zinc: when the body is deficient, it cannot be tasted, but when the body is saturated a metallic, acidic and unpleasant taste occurs. Therefore, an easy way to determine your own need is to purchase Zinc lozenges, available where vitamins are sold, and designed to ease sore throats. It's best to get a low potency (about 5 mg) with a minimum of other agents. By counting the lozenges and taking note of when the taste changes one can, after a few days, roughly determine your body's need for Zinc. 15 mg per day is certainly a safe dose for most adults. Because minerals accumulate in the system (they are not water soluble) this amount will safely guard against any depletion, and meet the body's daily requirements. Considering the definite link between Zinc deficiency and prostate problems it is a supplement that most men should be taking. Rich food sources of Zinc include fish and seafoods (especially oysters), legumes, egg yolks, mushrooms, pumpkin seeds, sunflower seeds, soybeans, and nutritional yeasts. Among the richest plant sources of Zinc are oats (which are also very high in Silica, an important trace mineral, mentioned further on.) protein, polyunsaturated fats, fiber, and a good range of vitamins and minerals.

Sulfur has been referred to as nature's 'beauty mineral' because of its' function in keeping hair glossy and smooth, and the complexion clear and youthful. Making up .25 of human body weight, Sulfur is stored in every cell of the body. The highest concentrations are found in the hair, skin, and nails. Sulfur is also part of the chemical structure of the amino acids L-Methionine, L-Cysteine, L-Taurine, and L-Glutathione. It disinfects the blood, and helps to protect the body against the harmful effects of radiation and pollution, thereby slowing down the aging process and increasing life span. Sulfur is present in Keratin, the tough protein substance that comprises most of the hair shaft. Folklore sometimes offers that an onion a day will prevent hair loss, and sure enough, onion is one of the richest food sources of Sulfur. In fact, many researchers believe that the wide range of health benefits attributed to garlic, and now similarly to the onion are largely due to the Sulfur containing nutrients of these foods. Large amounts of Sulfur are also found in dried beans, egg yolks, cabbage, brussel sprouts, fish, and turnips. In order to supplement with Sulfur it is necessary to acquire it as a single amino acid, and not as part of an amino complex.

Two other minerals to consider briefly are Potassium and Iron. Potassium is involved in regulating the transfer of nutrients to cells, and is required for hormonal secretions. Important to a healthy nervous system and a regular heart rhythm, Potassium aids in proper muscle contraction and works with Sodium to regulate the body's water balance. Potassium levels are depleted and disrupted by diuretic drugs and excess coffee consumption (caffeine is a mild diuretic). Constant fatigue is one of the symptoms of potassium deficiency. Hair-related symptoms to look for (aside from hair loss) are: lackluster hair, itchy scalp, dandruff, straw-like hair that is unmanageable and mats up, and hair that alternates between extremes of oily and dry. Potassium-rich food sources include avocados, bananas, molasses, dried fruits, nuts, potatoes, yams, and nutritional yeast.

Dry, brittle hair is one of the symptoms of a low grade Iron deficiency, as is general fatigue, rough and chapped skin, and ridges that run along the length or breadth of the fingernails. Hair loss itself is a symptom of full blown anemia. A suspected Iron deficiency is easy to confirm through a blood test obtained from your doctor. If you do decide to supplement with iron, do not use Ferrous Sulfate. This type, most commonly sold in pharmacies is not just constipating, but extremely difficult for the body to utilize. Non-utilized minerals do not wash through the body, but actually accumulate in the system. In the case of Iron, the accumulation occurs in the liver, potentially leading to liver problems. One should purchase Iron (and indeed all supplements) from a knowledgeable source. The safest and most effective Iron supplement on the market is called 'Floradix', available in both liquid and pill form. Good food sources include green leafy vegetables, eggs, fish, poultry, whole grains, almonds, beets, molasses, kidney and lima beans, dried prunes, dates, raisins, and the sweetener 'Sucanat'.

Our final mineral, Silica, is one that we shall devote abundant space to, as it is perhaps the most dramatic of all at stemming hair loss. It is important to note that we are talking about hair loss of a particular kind. We must differentiate between hair loss, per se, and what amounts to hair breakage. Have a look at some of the hairs on your pillow in the morning, or in your hair brush. Hair that is falling out will have a tiny white bulb at the end of it. Broken hair will not. The white bulb is not the hair root, but is the part of the hair nearest the root with some shed scalp skin or follicle lining attached. Since the root can't come out the possibility for re-growth always exists. In the case of breakage supplementation with Silica is the most effective means of rebuilding and strengthening the hair. Of course, in most cases the hair loss is a combination of both falling and breakage. However, the elimination of breakage is often half the battle, and the easiest part to accomplish.

Silicon is the second most abundant element in the earth's crust (oxygen being the first), where it is found mainly in the form of Silica, or $SiO2$. Silica is found in the stalks of grains and grasses, and is what gives these plants the ability to stand up against the wind. Some studies from the Soviet Union revealed a slowing of hair loss with Silica supplementation, noting that male skin with a weak growth of hair usually proved to have less Silica than male skin with a strong hair growth.

Silica stimulates cell metabolism and formation, inhibiting the aging process. We use it to maintain and repair our nails, hair, skin, teeth, eyes, and cell walls. The pancreas, thymus, thyroid, and coronary arteries are all rich in Silica. It increases bone calcium absorption, as well as collagen levels, making the bones harder and more flexible. This can occur even in the elderly, and in women past menopause, though it is commonly believed that it is not possible for these groups to rebuild bone. The Silicon content of mucopolysaccharides is extremely high. As mentioned in the previous chapter mucopolysaccharides are natural substances produced by the body that work with collagen as a tissue connector, so all connective and elastic tissues in their healthy state are rich in Silica.. However, as the levels of Silica decrease with age these tissues degenerate correspondingly. Declining Silica contents in human aortic tissues correlate very closely with a decline in the elasticity in the of the aortic vessel wall. It is not unusual for atherosclerotic arteries to contain as much as fourteen times less Silica than healthy arteries.

Because most of our foods are either over-processed or have been grown in soils subjected to demineralization (due to top soil erosion and continued use of incomplete chemical fertilizers) most of the foods we eat are Silica deficient. The richest source of Silica accessible to humans lies in the herb horsetail. The premium supplements to use are prepared through an aqueous, or water extract method from this herb. That said, never take a Silica related supplement that is made from unprocessed horsetail. Ingesting it straight, ground and tabulated, or encapsulated can have toxic side effects. This can not only destroy Vitamin B-1 in the body, but can seriously irritate the digestive tract. One herbal text reports that horsetail extract also helps reduce BPH, or inflammation of the prostate. Considering the link between Male Pattern Baldness and prostate problems this is another argument for the use of this supplement. Purchase your product in a health food or vitamin store, talk to someone who understands the difference, and make sure the label refers to "organic vegetal silica from aqueous extract".

Another commonly used form of Silica is a gel derived from quartz crystals. Described as a 'colloidal' preparation, it is a solution of particles suspended in water.

There are few supplements that can compare to Silica, both for preserving hair and for prolonging general youthfulness of the body. The daily requirement for the average adult is between 10 and 20 mg. The therapeutic dosage (as would be required to quickly retard hair breakage) is two to three times that amount for up to a month, then one would reduce to a maintenance dose. Rice is particularly high in Silica (remember the Chinese, East Indians, and Japanese, with their healthy hair and rice based diets?) as are oats. Other foods high in Silica include lettuce, parsnips, asparagus, onion, cucumber, strawberry, leek, cabbage, sunflower seeds, swiss chard, celery, rhubarb, and cauliflower.

Interestingly, soluble Silica can also strengthen the hair externally, perhaps accounting for the time-tested success of Nettle hair lotions. Nettle is another extremely rich source of Silica. Organic vegetal Silica, which is available as a supplement in powder form as well as capsules, will completely dissolve, so you can easily add it to your regular shampoo. This will stimulate healthier hair growth, strengthen the hair shaft, and assure beautiful shine and luster. There are one or two Silica containing shampoos currently on the market, but considering the expense of properly isolated Silica one must wonder if there is a sufficient amount in commercial shampoo to accomplish anything dramatic. To prepare your own concoction simply dissolve two tablespoons of powdered vegetal Silica extract in a few ounces of hot water, then pour into your shampoo bottle and agitate the mixture.

To obtain optimum mineralization from your diet you should remember that all foods recommended in this and other sections must be organically grown in order to guarantee the level of nutrients. If a mineral is not in the soil it will not be in the food. Even though a plant may take over a dozen minerals from the soil modern fertilizing techniques rarely add more than a few back to it (nitrogen, phosphorus, and potassium). The soil eventually becomes depleted of all other minerals, and the plants no longer supply concentrated levels of these nutrients. Whole grains, seeds, and nuts are the best sources for minerals, along with fresh leafy and root vegetables, fresh fruits, and freshly made juices. These foods should be the basis of your daily fare. In choosing a mineral supplement to cover all the bases, as opposed to focusing on single elements, try to find one as complex and naturally occurring in form as possible. It should contain trace minerals, along with the primary ones, balanced by nature, not by scientific guesswork.

CHAPTER SEVEN

Essential Fatty Acids

MOST OF US are now aware that vitamins and minerals are essential for the growth and maintenance of a healthy body, but many are unaware of the implications of Essential Fatty Acids (EFAs— previously known as Vitamin F) as an essential third component. EFA deficiency may be as common as to be present in seventy-five per cent of terminal diseases leading to premature death, including cancer, heart disease, and diabetes.

EFAs, which keep the body, mind and emotions operating at a high level of wellness are referred to as 'essential' since they are not produced by the human body. They must, therefore, be part of the food supply. Some of the recognizable symptoms of low level deficiency are dry, brittle hair, hair loss, and skin problems ranging from itching and flaking to psoriasis. In more severe cases the symptoms elevate to fatigue, confusion, general weakness, easy bruising, pain, inflammation, and swelling of the joints. In examples of growing animals totally deprived of EFAs, there was in addition to hair loss and eczema an excessive thickening of the sebaceous glands. This is the strongest link between a lack of EFAs and hair loss. Two Japanese researchers, Masumi Inaba and Yoshikata Inaba, recently posited the 'Sebaceous Gland Hypothesis'. Their observations revealed that the excess sebum that often accompanies hair loss is the result of an enlargement of the sebaceous gland which is attached to each hair follicle. The enlarged gland increases sebum production, leading to clogging of the pores and malnutrition of the hair root, as well as raising the level of 5-alpha reductase. (See Chapter 2: Causes of Hair Loss) These researchers, from Inaba Aesthetic Surgery in Tokyo, believe that diet is a more probable cause of this condition than heredity. They noticed that prior to the introduction of animal fat into their diet after WW2 , Japanese hair was thick and healthy, with small sebaceous glands and little scalp oil. It has been noted in western research that thinning hair is often preceded by problems with greasy hair. In conjunction with the fact that EFAs have a normalizing effect on sex hormone response (including both estrogen and testosterone), and the link between these hormones, Benign Prostatic Hyperplasia and Male Pattern Baldness, the argument for EFA supple-mentation becomes very strong.

The supplemental sources of EFAs are Evening Primrose Oil, Flaxseed Oil, Wheat Germ Oil, Cod Liver Oil, and the oils from various other deep cold water fish. Eating deep water fish such as salmon, mackerel, trout, herring, or sardines two or three times a week can provide a reasonable amount of EFAs. Do not rely on Cod Liver Oil for EFAs. In order to obtain therapeutic amounts through this source one would run the risk of overdosing on Vitamins A and D. Salmon oil is a commercially available alternative fish oil, but the prime sources most often prescribed are Evening Primrose and Flax Oils. The two oils cover a slightly different range of Fatty Acids. In Europe, Flax Oil is used in cancer therapy, and for controlling blood pressure and cholesterol levels.

Evening Primrose Oil has been the subject of many studies. It is known to help prevent the hardening of the arteries, and aids in treating heart disease, premenstrual syndrome and multiple sclerosis. It is also used in treating cirrhosis of the liver and in relieving pain and inflammation. Although the distinction between Flax and Evening Primrose Oils is important to those with serious ailments, it is a subject beyond the scope of this book. As a supplement in treating hair loss, as well as for general health maintenance, it is best to take both oils. They may be taken (with food) alternately or together. Both come in capsule form, and Flax Oil is also available in bottles. The maintenance dosage of either oil is three capsules/ one tablespoon per day; while the therapeutic dosage is six capsules per day (or three of each). Because both of these oils are extracted from their natural media, they lack the co-factors necessary for assimilation. As such certain nutrients (including Biotin, Niacin, B-6, C, E, and Zinc) must be taken with them at the same time. The simplest way to achieve this is to take a multi-vitamin and mineral supplement.

Excess saturated fat in the diet competes with EFAs and actually exacerbates the effect of an EFA deficiency, so avoid taking the supplements with a meal high in such fats. Other factors that interfere with the body's utilization of EFAs include old age, diabetes, excessive alcohol, nutritional deficiencies, high cholesterol levels, persistent viral infections and the consumption of trans-fatty acids. Trans-fatty acids are formed by 'bad oils'—that is, vegetable oils which have been hydrogenated (to remain solid at room temperature, e.g. margarine), allowed to become rancid, or heated to high temperatures repeatedly (as in the case of deep fried food). Since good oils were, until recently, almost impossible to come by, bad oils were consumed excessively. This combination has lead to widespread deficiency of EFAs. It should be noted that trans-fatty acids are also responsible for free radical formation in the body. Free radicals are now believed to be responsible for the mechanisms of cancer, heart disease, immune system breakdown and premature aging. Free radicals are combated by anti-oxidants. Some of these are produced in the body; some are ingested in the form of nutrients (the most common being Beta-carotene, Vitamin C and Vitamin E).

Juices

THE LITERATURE of the natural foods movement abounds with information on reducing and reversing hair loss, much of it based on juice recipes. When the health food movement began some decades ago vitamin and mineral supplement pills were not available. Those pioneers in nutritional research and medicine found that the easiest and most effective way to provide the body with high levels of nutrients was to juice organic fruits and vegetables. In this form the specific nutrients of the plant are condensed, requiring little energy to be digested. These juices are readily assimilable by the body, and as bonded in structure (bound to co-factors) as regular food. One of the important benefits of juice is its high enzyme content, which not only helps in digesting the juice itself, but is also stored by the body for future use in digesting cooked foods, which lack enzymes. In order to capitalize on the enzyme content the juice must be made and consumed freshly. The longer a juice is stored the more the nutrients deteriorate, the enzymes going first, the minerals last. Bottled juices will provide minerals, and perhaps some vitamins, but having usually been pasteurized to prolong shelf life, are devoid of enzymes. Following are the most commonly recommended juices for hair loss problems. Most of the foods mentioned can be used interchangeably in recipes of your own devising. These formulations are all based on vegetable juices. However, should you wish to experiment with fruit juices remember that for optimal digestion and assimilation they should be ingested separately. Based on human digestive cycles, fruit juices are best taken in the morning, and vegetable juices in the afternoon. Of course, all the mineral and vitamin rich foods suggested for juicing may also be incorporated into the daily diet as whole foods, to great benefit.

In the fifties Dr. H. Kirschner had a reputation for reversing hair loss with his program of mineral supplementation. For the most part the minerals were extracted from freshly squeezed vegetable juices. Based on the principle of furnishing food to the scalp nerves and roots of the hair via the bloodstream his most frequently used treatment was carrot juice. Organic carrot juice contains most of the minerals required by the body, and is rich in Silica, Sulfur, Iron, and Potassium. It also creates an alkaline balance in the bloodstream, strengthens the nervous system, and works on the endocrine glandular system to help issue valuable hormones needed by the hair roots. Carrot juice is enhanced by the addition of cucumber, which, due to its' high Silica and Sulfur content is recommended for the promotion of hair growth. Cucumber also contains Vitamins A, B-Complex, and C, as well as Calcium, Manganese, Phosphorus, Potassium, and Sodium. Sodium is a balanced constituent of food and should be of no worry to you if your blood pressure is okay. Damaging levels of sodium come from table salt, processed foods, and excess meat consumption. In fact, the sodium content of both cucumber and lettuce, also frequently recommended, actually assists in maintaining the calcium in the vegetable, keeping it in constant solution until it is utilized by the body. Lettuce is also rich in Silica and Vitamin A.

Spinach juice is frequently advised, both in combination with lettuce juice, or in a lettuce and carrot combination. Those with a history of kidney stones should avoid spinach, as it contains a large amount of oxalic acid, a substance commonly implicated in the formation of stones. Non-organic spinach, it should be added, is notorious for its high pesticide content..

Alfalfa juice, in combination with lettuce and carrot juice, is a formulation mentioned repeatedly in the literature concerning the growth of new hair, and restoration of its' original color. The Arabs, recognizing its' superior level of nutrients and corresponding health benefits named it "Al Falfa", meaning the "Father of All Foods". Alfalfa's nutrient content is so high because its' roots burrow deep into clean, unused earth (as deep as thirty feet), reaching minerals inaccessible to other plants. Rich in Vitamins A, B's (including Biotin, Inositol, and PABA) C, D, E, K, and U, alfalfa has high amounts of the minerals Calcium, Iron Potassium, Phosphorus, Magnesium, Silica, and Sulfur, as well as trace minerals. High in protein and chlorophyll (which helps detoxify the bloodstream and build red blood cells), alfalfa is also a source of eight enzymes which are known to help metabolize and assimilate nutrients. It is important to make the distinction here between alfalfa the plant, which is not commercially available as a foodstuff, and alfalfa the sprout, which is. The sprout, unable to send shoots deep into the earth, is not known to have the same qualities as the plant. Therefore, the accessible means of obtaining alfalfa is to purchase tablets at your health food store. Make sure they come from organic alfalfa. Like Kelp tablets, six to ten per day are necessary to receive any noticeable benefits.

Nettles are also very beneficial when used in juices, for they are extremely high in Silica, Iron, and Potassium, and also rich in Iodine, Sulfur, and Vitamins A and C. While fresh nettles may be difficult for you to come by, the dried product is easily purchased, and may be brewed as a tea for daily intake.

Since the time of the Roman Empire watercress was believed effective at reversing falling hair. We now know that healthy hair growth is partially dependent on the Sulfur bearing amino acids. Watercress contains more Sulfur than any other vegetable, excluding horseradish. It also contains Vitamins A and C, B-1, Folic Acid, Biotin, B-3, Pantotheic Acid, and the minerals Potassium, Calcium, Sodium, Iron, and Zinc. It is one of the best sources of Iodine.

The juice of the watercress is much too strong to take alone, so try as handful of it along with four or five carrots., half a handful of parsley, a couple stalks of celery, and perhaps some lettuce. Spinach is overpoweringly strong in combination with watercress. Another strongly flavored juice, to be added judiciously, is parsnip, which contains the winning combination of Sulfur and Silica in high amounts, as well as Potassium and Phosphorus. Adding a quarter inch thick slice of raw ginger root to four or five juiced carrots, along with a few other choice vegetables will give both the juice and your circulation some zing.

CHAPTER NINE

Circulation

MAINTAINING A HEALTHY HEAD OF HAIR depends in part on the quality and quantity of circulation to the hair roots. If the blood, lymph, oxygen and nutrient supply to any given hair follicle is cut off it will die. Whatever the cause, this is the process that begins hair loss and leads to baldness. The most common and easily remedied cause is tension. Excess stress affects our minds and bodies. It tightens muscles, causes skin problems such as eczema, and reduces blood flow to the extremities. As a result of the muscular contraction which accompanies tension, tightened blood vessels constrict the capillaries feeding hair follicles and the hair roots become starved. Stress-induced loss of circulation can work in conjunction with a stressed hormonal system (specifically the androgenic hormones produced by stressed adrenal glands) to create a scalp that is prone to severe hair loss. Due to thinner scalp tissue men are more prone to baldness as a result of stress than women.

Another cause of reduced circulation is seborrhea of the scalp. This disorder of the oil secreting sebaceous glands is akin to a less common form of dandruff that involves the formation of greasy or crusty scales on the scalp (The most common form of dandruff is the dry, flaky type, and is not linked to hair loss). In both these cases excess sebum (oily secretions) combines with dead cell flakes from normal sloughing, clogging the follicles and inhibiting the hair reproduction cycle. Dry hair will often accompany this syndrome because the oily flakes clogging the follicles prevent oil from traveling down the hair shaft. When sebum combines with excessive scalp perspiration it can form hard, crystalline follicle plugs. This causes follicle congestion and tissue hardening which inhibits nutrient flow to the hair. Apple cider vinegar and jojoba oil can be especially helpful with these types of problems.

Arthritis or tightness in the neck and spine can tighten blood vessels in the head, reducing circulation and blood flow. Body massage is an excellent way of relieving tension and tightness. Physical activity will also reduce stress and increase blood flow to the extremities, including the head and scalp. Common sense dictates that we must not only reduce circulatory inhibitors and increase general circulation, but must also dramatically increase blood flow to the very top of the head. There are several effective methods of accomplishing this.

For those who like devices, both the 'Back Swing' and 'Gravity Inversion Boots' (used to hang upside down) will bring greatly increased blood flow to the scalp. However, the boots are only for the very fit, whereas the swing may be used by most everyone, except those with very high blood pressure or other serious circulatory disorders. In either case use should begin very gradually, and increased slowly.

Two low tech, inexpensive options are the slant board and the headstand. The slant board should be used at roughly a forty five degree angle, working up to fifteen minutes a day. The headstand, a well known Yoga practice, is even more effective than the slant board. There are those of the opinion that this is the single most important thing one can do to prevent hair loss and improve the health of your hair. Work up to two to three minutes, twice a day. Inversion techniques, with the added bonus of increasing the mental faculties by increasing blood and oxygen flow to the brain are even more effective when backed up with massage techniques.

Finger massage is a very efficient way to improve blood circulation in the scalp. However, because it is essential to keep the blood circulating constantly, massaging once or twice a week will not accomplish much. Ideally, scalp massage should be performed at least twice a day in order to be beneficial. Try to include it as part of your hair washing regimen, as a way of working it into regular habit. Place all ten fingertips firmly on the head and, without moving the fingers, push the whole scalp in a circular motion for a few seconds. Then, moving from front to back, and then back to front, place the fingers in a new position and repeat. Cover the whole scalp, including the temples, forehead, and neck, where you may also use an upward pushing motion. Avoid rubbing the problem area, as this could break hairs at the surface and traumatize the follicles.

Some experts allow for a flat handed scalp massage, placing the palm of the hand against the scalp and rotating, as an alternative to the finger massage. It will loosen the tightness of the scalp, relaxing without damaging any hair but, while it is easier to do, it is not as effective as the finger technique. An effective scalp massage may also be attained using an electric vibrator. The better models have

How Hair is Nourished

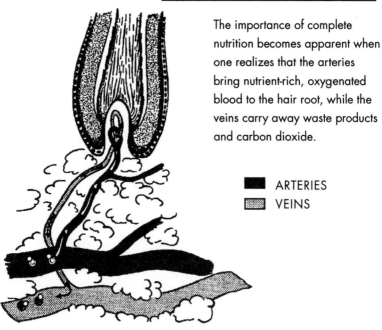

The importance of complete nutrition becomes apparent when one realizes that the arteries bring nutrient-rich, oxygenated blood to the hair root, while the veins carry away waste products and carbon dioxide.

■ ARTERIES
▨ VEINS

an attachment designed for scalp massage, and are easy to use offering an effortless massage. At the very least use it twice a day for about five to eight minutes, and use a similar motion to that of the finger massage.

An Oriental circulatory technique (based on Qi Kung) involves the ancient art of raising and circulating body energies. Place your fingers at the center of the base of your skull and bring them to each ear, tapping them gently about thirty times. Repeat this exercise about eight times, beginning a little higher on the skull each time until you reach the crown of your head. This is designed to bring blood to the scalp and face, nourishing the hair and giving the skin a youthful glow.

CHAPTER TEN

Herbs and Plants, External Use

CERTAIN NATIVE AMERICAN TRIBES had a remedy for graying or falling hair that involved the common grape vine: In the spring they would cut off the end of a branch, tie a gourd onto it and collect the sap. The sap was then applied generously and worked into the scalp and roots of the hair. An alternative method was to make a tea of the roots of the grape vine. This was used as a wash two or three times a month when graying or falling hair first became apparent, and then used only once a month, once the problem was under control.

Few of us today would go to such effort. Yet every culture has had its' own approach to the problem of hair loss, based both on the variety of indigenous plants available and its' cultural perspective. Let's look at a few of the more improbable ancient techniques before approaching those with a stronger historical and scientific base.

From the "De Material Medica" of the famous Greek herbalist

of the first century AD, Dioscorides: "Wild olive oil will not only prevent hair from falling out but will also prevent it from turning gray...intended to be rubbed into the scalp daily."

From the "Ebers Papyrus", and Egyptian medical document, four thousand years old: (1) "mix together the fat of a lion, fat of a hippopotamus, fat of a crocodile, fat of a cat, fat of a serpent, and fat of a Nubian ibex, and rub the mixture on the head. (2) Mix the crushed flax seed with an equal quantity of oil, add water from a well, and rub mixture on the head."

Aztec remedies: (1) Make a poultice of Nettles, serpents, scorpions, and millipedes that have been ground up and boiled together. (2) For hair that will not grow, bathe the head with morning water (urine) from a woman who is with child."

It is easy to laugh at such remedies when we look at them from the modern perspective, but these were thriving and successful civilizations. One out of two of their members did not die of heart disease, nor did one out of four die of cancer, as do members of our own civilization. Perhaps we would do well then, to look a little closer at the remedies and techniques of bygone peoples and cultures, as well as at our own folklore. Before leaving these examples let's consider: olive oil and flax oil both provide essential fatty acids, recently proven to be necessary for healthy hair growth. To this day, people of Greek or Mediterranean descent apply virgin olive oil to their hair and scalp to improve hair condition. Nettles are one of the most common herbs used in natural hair loss remedies around the world. Science has recently found some success in reversing hair loss with the topical application of synthetic estrogen; its natural analog is prevalent in the urine of a pregnant woman.

As mentioned, Nettles have been used as a hair growth stimulant for centuries. They are rich in vitamins A and C, and a wide range of minerals including Iodine, Silicon, and Sulfur, all especially good for the hair. The other two herbs frequently mentioned in herbal texts and folklore are Rosemary, both for cleansing the scalp and stimulating the hair root, and Sage, which is claimed to not only stop falling hair, but to strengthen and thicken the hair shaft. Two remedies which use all three herbs are:

(1) Boil together in water rosemary, sage, peach leaf, nettle and burdock. Strain and use to wash hair daily. (2) Steep one ounce of ground rosemary, two ounces of ground sage, and half an ounce of ground nettles in one pint of ethyl alcohol for a week. Strain, and

add one ounce of olive oil, one ounce of castor oil, and one ounce of water. Shake before using as a hair lotion, either before bed or at least fifteen minutes before shampooing.

Apple cider vinegar is frequently mentioned in folk remedies for hair loss. It is reputed to have a normalizing effect on the scalp's oil glands and pH level. More importantly, its' high acidity and powerful enzymes destroy harmful bacteria responsible for several scalp conditions. Disturbances in the scalp's epidermal cell renewal can cause an accumulation of dead cells at the skin's surface. Excessive oil gland activity causes the scale like dead cells to become more firmly attached to the scalp and each other. This forms a breeding ground for the harmful bacteria called 'bottle bacillus'. Itching and dandruff ensue, and hair follicles become clogged. Deprived of natural oils, hair begins to break off or fall out. The benefits of apple cider vinegar can be obtained as follows: Part hair into sections. Apply two tablespoons directly to the scalp with a moistened cotton ball. Allow between fifteen minutes and three hours before shampooing. In acute cases this can be repeated on a daily basis. An after-shampoo rinse, suitable for the whole body, uses one third of a cup of vinegar per quart of rinse water.

An old English herbal text suggests washing the head once a day with strong, warm sage tea, and using diluted apple cider vinegar as a rinse, to check the falling hair and stimulate growth.

Another old herbal recipe is to make a strong decoction by mixing fresh, dry nettles with equal amounts of water and apple cider vinegar, then simmering it down until it resembles the color of coffee. This is rubbed into the scalp once a day (the book also recommends washing the scalp each morning with cold water, a great aid to circulation).

One interesting nettle formula for hair loss includes onion: one part Nettle leaves, one part onion, one part seventy per cent alcohol. Soak the leaves and onion in the alcohol for several days, then massage into the scalp before washing the hair, in order to stimulate hair growth. This is simple, inexpensive remedy comes from a highly respected source, Dr. A Vogel, a Swiss herbalist known throughout the world. At the time he wrote this in 1952 there was, on the European market, a deodorized onion scalp lotion.

Essential oils distilled from plants and herbs are an effective remedy for a wide range of hair and scalp ailments. They add luster and shine to the hair and increase circulation to the scalp. In addition, they are easily absorbed into the lower levels of the skin, where new cells are generated. Because essential oils are too strong to be applied directly to the skin they must be diluted with a carrier oil. Jojoba and olive oils are particularly well suited to this purpose. As a general rule ten drops of essential oil should be mixed with one ounce of carrier oil. Massage into the scalp for a minimum of fifteen minutes before shampooing. Some of the most commonly used essential oils for hair loss are Cedarwood, Clary Sage, Lavender, Eucalyptus and Rosemary. Clary Sage helps dissolve sebum deposits. Lavender regulates the acid mantle of the scalp and gives body and shine to the hair shaft. Eucalyptus regulates sebum, reduces inflammation of the scalp, and is a deep cleaning agent. Rosemary shares much in common with Lavender. Most of these essential oils also stimulate circulation in the scalp. Another popular oil is Cajuput or Tea Tree Oil, which is especially good for severe dandruff, and is also an effective disinfectant and bactericide.

Jojoba (pronounced ho-ho-ba) oil has been used by Mexican and desert Indian tribes for centuries to keep their hair healthy and to relieve skin problems such as dermatitis, eczema, and psoriasis. Jojoba oil resembles the skin's own natural sebum secretions, and so has a remarkable affinity for skin and hair. A perfect moisturizer for hypoallergenic skin, it is completely absorbed into the skin's deep layers. Jojoba oil removes sebum deposits which collect around the hair follicles, solidify and cause dandruff, hair loss, and scalp disorders. It also makes the scalp less acidic, and is great for both dry and oily hair, as well as itchy scalp problems. Jojoba contains B vitamins, vitamin E, Silicon, Chromium, Copper, Zinc, and is high in Iodine.

One of the herbal folk remedies to prove itself to modern researchers is the "Cayenne Pepper Hair Tonic.". A powerful skin irritant such as cayenne not only brings a good blood flow to the scalp, but also causes histamine release which stimulates cell division, encouraging new growth. The tonic recipe is as follows: Mix four ounces of cayenne pepper with one pint of one hundred proof vodka (or pure alcohol diluted with twenty per cent distilled water). Let stand for two weeks, shaking the mixture once each day. Strain through several layers of fine cloth or a nylon stocking until the mixture is free of pepper. Once or twice a day rub a small amount onto the thinning or balding areas of the scalp. Avoid contact with the eyes. Effects should be noticeable within five weeks.

Another hair growth tonic that stimulates circulation to the scalp, but is simpler to prepare and use, involves juicing a one to two inch piece of ginger root (you may find this easier to do if you grate it first). Just massage the juice into your scalp and let it dry for ten or fifteen minutes, then shampoo. This will create a distinct tingling sensation.

Certain Indian tribes of Mexico claim that their thick, healthy hair, resistant to graying and balding, is due in part to their regular use of the gel from the Aloe Vera plant. They rub the gel into the hair and scalp, and leave it on overnight. The next morning it is washed out without the use of any other cleansing product, such as soap or shampoo, as certain properties of the plant produce a low sudsing action. The plant has been used in the past and present for a number of ailments including arthritis, burns, insect bites, cold sores, dry skin, and internally for ulcers and hiatal hernias. Aloe Vera was recently studied by the Japanese (now more prone to baldness as they disregard traditional ways and adopt western eating habits) for its' potential to prevent hair loss. It has shown some success at reducing hair loss. Aside from containing an abundance of amino acids, vitamins, and minerals, Aloe Vera also has the ability to balance the skins' pH level. Its proteolytic enzymes help to slough off dead skin cells and open pores. Due to its lignins and polysaccharides, it also allows other ingredients to penetrate more easily and deeply into the skin. One key mucopolysaccharide, known as Acemannan, is most highly concentrated in aloe products made from the whole leaf. Acemannan interjects itself into cell membranes, causing an increase in the membrane's fluidity and permeability. This facilitates the outward flow of toxins and the inward flow of nutrients to and from the cell. The highest quality Aloe Vera products are those which use the whole leaf (as opposed to just the inside of the leaf) and which offer standardized mucopolysaccharide levels. Aloe also works especially well for drawn and painful scalp conditions, with the advantage of remaining unnoticeable even if used throughout the day.

From India comes this recipe for a shampoo designed to stimulate hair growth: Combine and mix seventy per cent Aloe Vera gel, twenty per cent wheat germ oil, and ten per cent coconut milk. Wet hair, apply shampoo and massage into scalp. Leave on for five minutes, then rinse.

Above we have detailed the herbs and plants most commonly referred to in the literature on and the subject of hair loss. Following are some random elements mentioned only rarely or in isolation. They are included for those using this book as a reference.

Ginseng root used as lotion in an alcohol base is mentioned both in Chinese literature, and is a component of 'Formula 101 Hair Liniment', sold in sixteen countries around the world.

Walnut meat is also a component of 'Formula 101', and, next to flax seed oil, is the richest vegetable source of omega 3 essential fatty acids. From Europe comes this "Walnut Leaf Hair Loss Lotion." Cover two heaping teaspoons of finely chopped walnut leaves with one cup of boiling water, cover and steep, then strain. massage into the scalp daily. The same steps done with marshmallow leaves is also recommended as a remedy.

Nicholas Culpepper (1617–1654), the famous English herbalist offered this solution: Use four ounces of crushed ripe peach pits in one pint of vinegar. Apply three times per day. Here we assume he is referring to apple cider vinegar, and that the formulation must be allowed to sit for a week or two, and then strained.

While many will choose not to go through the trouble of making their own lotions and tonics, both the raw ingredients mentioned in this chapter and hair loss products containing many of these substances are available in health food stores and herbal shops. At very least, these are ingredients to look for when choosing shampoos, conditioners and other hair care products.

Hormonal Remedies

Various hormonal remedies have been somewhat effective at countering Male Pattern Baldness, (a hormonal affliction). However, they are not without their limitations. Typically, they are effective at preventing hair loss, but not as effective at re-growth. In addition, topical applications can easily enter the bloodstream, and, as these are hormonal drugs, can upset the body's delicate balance.

The topical application of female hormones to the scalp has displayed some success at inhibiting DHT formation by blocking its' receptors (as does a testosterone compound salve). However, hair re growth averages only about ten per cent, and in some cases it was more than a year before any noticeable effects were observed.

A safer alternative is "Wild Yam Cream," which contains three per cent natural progesterone. Progesterone is a hormone that provides the building block for all steroid hormones. It has the same nucleus as estrogen and performs similar functions.The cream is sold by naturopaths and in health food stores. It is used to safely and naturally raise a woman's estrogen levels in order to retain and deposit calcium into her bone mass. It also helps in dealing with symptoms of menopause, helping to forgo the need for synthetic estrogen therapy.The cream base contains a delivery system to carry both through the skin and into the bloodstream, in order to penetrate sufficiently into the scalp.

Sarsaparilla Extract was discovered in 1939, and is sold under its' Latin name, Similax Officianalus. It contains hormonal compounds similar in structure to testosterone. For this reason it is ingested mostly by athletes seeking to raise their testosterone levels.Available in health food and vitamin stores, the extract is in an alcohol base, which is an ideal delivery system for topical application.

More effective at promoting hair re-growth than topical hormone treatment is a substance called Polysorbate 80. Research done at Finland's Helsinki University claimed an eighty per cent success rate in both women and men, with no significant side effects (although there is an increase in hair loss for the first week or two, due to the loosening of hairs in the resting phase). Re-growth was reported in hundreds of men in their fifties and sixties who used Polysorbate 80 every day for a year.

Polysorbate 80 is approved by the FDA as a shampoo surfactant, and as a food additive.As a food additive it is used as an emulsifier; an agent that causes water and fats to mix. It is considered to be of negligible toxicity, and as such is found in everyday products such as mayonnaise, salad dressings, and some liquid detergents. It also the base of the 'Helsinki Formula', and most other commercial hair loss products designed for external use. Polysorbate 80 is said to work through removing DHT and cholesterol from the scalp, and causing the release of histamine (a cellular growth factor) in the scalp. Scientists using it were able to reverse a degree of early tissue disorganization occurring at the inception of some chemically induced cancers. As such, it may also affect the control of genetic activities in the hair follicle cells.

Pure Polysorbate 80 is commonly available in health food stores. To use it, coat the scalp with a thin film in the balding areas ten or fifteen minutes before shampooing. It is a viscous substance, so place several drops on various areas of the scalp, then rub the drops in and around vigorously.The scalp should redden and feel slightly warm, due to the histamine release. Pure Polysorbate 80 washes out easily, though if you get it in your eyes it will be mildly irritating, just like any shampoo. If it is going to work for you, you will notice thin, short hairs within two or three months of daily use. After a longer period the hairs should improve in quality and quantity.

CHAPTER ELEVEN

Devices and Gadgets

A 1989 STUDY at the University of British Columbia indicated much potential for arresting hair loss through electric pulses to the scalp. Dr. Stuart Maddin, a dermatologist with UBC's Adult Hair Clinic gave thirty men fifteen minutes of electric pulses once a week, through a hair dryer like device. By the end of the thirty six week study all but one of the subjects had either increased hair growth or reduced unnatural loss. The study found that 'electrotrichogenesis' could increase the numbers of hairs on balding men's heads by up to sixty-six per cent. Similar electrical treatments are used to heal bone fractures, speed tissue healing, and remove skin ulcers and scar tissue. In this case the device alters the electromagnetic field around the hair follicles, changing the protein synthesis in the cells. Though the treatment has been approved by the Federal Health Protection Branch in Canada, and is being examined by the FDA in the US. Dr. Maddin is unsure whether it will ever become a commercially available treatment.

In 1987 two Canadian entrepreneurs approached the hair loss

problem from an unusual perspective: hand reflexology. Reflexology, considered akin to a western version of acupuncture is based on physically manipulating acupuncture points on the hands and feet, using the practitioners thumbs and fingers rather than needles. Reflexologist Mildred Carter, in her book on hand reflexology highly recommends fingernail buffing for follicle stimulation and healthy hair. She refers to testimonials of new growth, color change, and the prevention of graying. At least one disease of the scalp, Alopecia Areata, which can cause complete hair loss, also produces pitted finger nails.

The 'Hair Tech' was designed to provide an easy method of nail stimulation in the comfort of your home. It weighs in at six pounds, and measures twelve by four inches. A limited study was run with the new device. Thirty men between the ages of nineteen and fifty nine received a once a day ten minute buffing of their finger nails. Within six weeks those experiencing excessive hair loss were noting a dramatic improvement. After approximately three months on the program various claims were being made by the subjects including: improved hair condition, new visible growth, natural color returning, looser scalp, and faster growth of finger nails. While results varied from person to person, every subject reported that they had stopped losing excessive amounts of hair. It should be pointed out that the study was performed by the 'Hair Tech' company. Nonetheless, they offer a guarantee that unnatural hair loss will stop within thirty days, otherwise they refund the cost of the product.

Magnetics are currently enjoying a resurgence in the Orient and Europe as therapy for a wide range of ailments including arthritis, muscular pain, and inflammatory conditions. One catalogue offers a 'Magnetic Therapy Brush' with 'Induction Bristles' (made from metal) to invigorate the main acupuncture points of the scalp, stimulating blood circulation. It is claimed that daily use will help prevent hair loss, dandruff, and seborrhea, while strengthening hair and promoting new growth. It also claims to relieve neck pain and stiffness.

It is worthy of note that finding even three or four reputable 'devices and gadgets' was a difficult task. This area, more than any other in the hair loss field, should be approached with caution. Look for impartial studies rather than 'personal testimonials', and always check your sources. Remember, a firm dietary base is your primary defense against hair loss. Devices and Gadgets should be considered complementary.

CHAPTER TWELVE

Choosing a Shampoo and Conditioner

EXCESSIVE SHAMPOOING, particularly with most commonly used commercial shampoos, can cause the hair to lose minerals such as Calcium, Phosphorus, Iron , and Nitrogen. This is due to the harsh chemicals present in most of these products. Not only will they damage your hair, but they can pose a threat to general health. Formaldehyde, which is used in shampoo as a preservative, is often disguised as 'Quanternium-15'. Aside from being carcinogenic at certain levels, it can prove to be an irritant to the skin, eyes, and respiratory system. Shampoos may also contain ammonia, coal tar colors, synthetic detergents, ethanol, and artificial fragrances. It's no wonder allergic reactions to these products are common.

It is safest to purchase your shampoo at a natural foods store, or from a professional at a hair salon. Make sure they can address your concerns about excess chemicals. Read the labels, and don't hesitate to ask questions. Try different shampoos until you find one that you like, then alternate to a different brand every so often. Remember, the shampoo you used in your twenties may not be the best choice in your forties. This is because hair, like skin, becomes drier as we age, producing less of the oil which serves as a protective shield for the hair shaft. Look for mild cleansers such as cocoamide betaine or cocoamido propyl betaine which are extracted from coconut, or sulfosuccinates, which are derived from wheat germ oil. Even Sodium Lauryl Sulfate, and other sulfates used in 'natural' shampoos, can strip away too much oil from the hair, leaving a film of shampoo residue. Layered shampoo residues, combined with excess sebum and perspiration salts, can cause follicles to plug. Because these sulfate surfactants are made in a process that uses sulfuric acid, they can become unstable, reverting back to sulfuric acid and irritating the skin, scalp and eyes. Protein or Keratin in shampoo will give hair body and bounce. By coating the hair, protein fills in gaps and pits in the damaged hair shaft, and temporarily repairs split ends by gluing the frayed ends back together. Hydrolyzed soy protein, containing amino propane sulfonic acid can reinforce the hair and, through regulating sebum production, can also stimulate growth.

One key ingredient to look for is Panthenol (pro-Vitamin B-5). Panthenol is used to improve hair strength and elasticity. It works because the molecule is small enough to actually work its way into the hair cortex, where it can bond to the building blocks of hair. Panthenol can strengthen undamaged hair by up to 20%. Damaged hair shows even more dramatic results. Also look for anti-oxidants such as Vitamins A, C, E, and nourishing herb and plant extracts including Aloe Vera, Burdock, Chamomile, Chaparral, Horsetail, Nettles, Rosemary, and Sage.

A properly balanced shampoo is 5.5 pH. (The acid range is from 0 to 7 pH, and the alkaline range is from 7.1 to 14.0 pH) A properly balanced shampoo, which is slightly acidic, does not coat the hair but leaves it shinier, and is gentle enough to use daily. A "body" shampoo is mildly alkaline, and though not harsh enough to be damaging, it tends to swell the hair shaft slightly.

Regular use of a conditioner is necessary to maintain healthy hair. A conditioner is best compared to a skin moisturizer. It is especially important for dry hair and hair overexposed to aggravating environmental conditions such as drying wind, heat, sunlight, and chemicals such as chlorine. Chlorine, for example, chemically bonds to hair, robbing it of moisture and leaving it dull, brittle, and susceptible to breakage. These environmental factors damage the hair shaft, not the follicle. As such, the condition is preventable. Conditioners coat the hair cuticle with a fine film which smoothes it and temporarily rebinds split ends back together, making the hair appear thicker. Conditioners also reduce static and restore softness, shine, and manageability.

As with shampoos look for a minimum of unrecognizable chemicals, and a clearly defined protein. Keratin or amino acids should be included (again, for filling in cracks and breaks in the hair shaft and gluing split ends back together). Check the label to ensure the inclusion of natural oils (unless you have excessively oily hair) such as Safflower, Jojoba, and Evening Primrose. These lubricate hair strands, reduce tangling, and prevent moisture loss. If your hair is oily, then check the label for a natural moisturizer called 'NaPCA'. NaPCA is found in human skin, and is not oil based. If you have extremely damaged hair you may wish to consider using a deep conditioner once a month. These are specialty products and must be left on for a minimum of ten minutes. One of the best and safest is the neutral 'henna', a natural clay in use since the time of the ancient Egyptians. Henna seals the cuticle, protecting hair and making it glossier. Periodic applications add additional protective coatings.

Currently on the market there are shampoos with built in conditioners. These are best avoided. Shampoo and conditioning serve two different functions, and by combining them the effectiveness of each is decreased. Anti-dandruff shampoos are among the most dangerous of all hair care products, the other leading two being aerosol hair spray and styling mousse. Dandruff shampoos use toxic medications to prevent the scalp from peeling. The most popular agent is selenium sulfide, which, taken in excess, has shown to cause degeneration of the liver and other organs. Dandruff shampoos may also contain toxic creosol and the carcinogenic 'polyvinyl pyrrlidone plastic' (PVP), not to mention the standard chemicals found in most commercial shampoos. While the FDA maintains that the quantities of these toxic substances in a shampoo poses no threat, it is important to remember that the skin and scalp are an avenue to the bloodstream, and that most carcinogens are cumulative.

One final word about dandruff: many people with serious dandruff problems maintain healthy hair throughout their lives. For those with thinning hair, however, a dandruff problem may worsen the condition. Dandruff itself does not cause baldness. It is the result of increased skin cell production (which is caused in part by excess protein intake) combined with excessive oil secretions. The two most basic steps in dealing with dandruff are massaging the scalp and brushing hair frequently. This dislodges dead cells. Frequent shampooing (with a mild shampoo that won't dry the scalp) also helps to rid the scalp of dead skin scales and oily secretions.

CHAPTER THIRTEEN

Washing, Drying, and Brushing

BEFORE ENTERING THE SHOWER or beginning to wash your hair give it a good brushing, and massage the scalp as well. These steps will loosen the dirt and scalp flakes, activate the oil glands, and encourage circulation. It is important to pre-rinse for at least one full minute before applying shampoo. This begins the removal of loosened debris from the scalp and facilitates better distribution of a smaller amount of shampoo. Using too much shampoo can leave the hair dull because the more used, the more difficult it becomes to completely remove when rinsing. Avoid using extremely hot water. This can actually increase temporary hair loss by softening the scalp and making it easier to pull hairs from their roots.

To apply shampoo, pour the minimum amount necessary onto the palm of your hand, rub your hands together and smooth the shampoo evenly over your hair. Do not pour shampoo directly on your hair as this saturates one spot to excess. Massage the shampoo into the scalp with the tips of the fingers (not the fingernails, which can irritate the scalp), spreading the lather and gently working the whole scalp area. Then rinse with warm water, and continue rinsing longer than you think is necessary. The ideal final rinsing should be with water moving progressively from cool to cold. Cold water will stimulate circulation and shrink the outer layer of the hair, making it smoother, shinier and more manageable. It also makes the hairs stiffer, stronger and locks them more firmly into their roots.

Some people need to wash their hair every day, some only once a week. Most fall in between these two extremes. How often one should shampoo depends on three factors. The first factor is the amount of oil your scalp naturally secretes. Signs of excessive scalp oil requiring more frequent shampooing include: dull and limp hair, itchy scalp, and greasy or oily looking hair that clings to the scalp. The second factor is your environment. If you live in a city with high levels of air pollution, then you will need to shampoo more frequently than someone living in a place with cleaner air. Finally, the season of the year is also a factor. During the heat of summer your head will perspire more than in cooler weather, and so requires more frequent washing. In cold, dry winter air your natural oil production may reduce to a point where shampooing is more seldom required.

For those who shampoo every day, and assuming that no unusual amounts of dirt and debris have been picked up, one washing should be sufficient. If those who shampoo less frequently choose to lather-up twice, it is recommended that they use a very mild shampoo. Buy one based on advice from a professional, either at a salon or a natural foods store. Labels can be misleading. A good shampoo will allow for deep cleaning without stripping the hair of its natural oils. When hair is "squeaky clean", it is probably over-cleaned. This is unnecessary and damaging to hair.

After the hair has been washed and thoroughly rinsed, apply the conditioner. Apply in a manner similar to that for the shampoo: pour a little into one palm, then rub the hands together and smooth it over the hair. However, remember that a conditioner is for the hair and not the scalp, so you need not work it into the scalp as you would with shampoo. Conditioners can be used as often as you shampoo, but don't use too much; you can overcondition your hair. Excess conditionings can weigh the hair down and reduce, instead of enhance, lustre and body. One with very fine hair may find that frequent use, or that certain brands may cause their hair to have a flat and limp look. Those with oily hair may find certain brands exacerbate the problem. The answer, as with shampoos, is trial and error. If your hair is not damaged you may opt to use a conditioner only once or twice a week. In any case most conditioners will have done their job within 30 seconds of application, so it is not really necessary to leave it on any longer than that.

After conditioning, squeeze or shake out excess water, and pat your hair dry using the towel as a blotter. Don't rub your hair or you may rough up the cuticle layer surface, or break fragile hair shafts. A hair style for which air drying will suffice is ideal; blowdryers can damage hair if improperly used. If you must use a blowdryer, do so after you have towel-dried the hair from wet to damp. Use a dryer with power less than 1000 watts, and set it at the lowest heat level. Stop as soon as the hair is dry (or even still slightly damp). Damage is done by over-drying. A wide nozzle dryer is preferable, as it diffuses the heat more and is easier on the hair. Keep the dryer at least six inches from the hair and keep it moving, directing the air over and through the hair. The nozzle should not be directed at the scalp and hair roots.

Hair that is wet or is being blow dried should be combed with a wide-toothed, smooth-edged comb with blunt tips. Hair swells on contact with water and becomes more fragile when wet. At this point the hair is so elastic that a brush may easily stretch and snap the hair shaft. Work out tangles by combing gently, starting from the ends and working toward the scalp.

Brushing

Regular brushing is an important step in your effort to prevent hair loss and improve the quality of your hair. The pulling effect of brushing aids circulation and stimulates the scalp. It also brings oil from the roots of the hair all the way down to the ends, promoting a more lustrous look. Finally, it helps to brush out debris such as dust, dirt and flakes of dandruff.

In order to achieve deep, scalp-stimulating brushing, you must work on your hair twice daily. Gently brush for three to five minutes, once in the morning and once in the evening. Brush for three minutes if your hair is short, and up to five minutes if it is longer.

Bending your head toward the floor while brushing will bring more blood flow to the head, increasing circulation to the scalp. Do not overbrush (your scalp should not feel raw and sore afterwards), or you'll risk causing 'traction alopecia', a condition of temporary hair loss as a result of overzealous brushing. Alternate with up and down strokes. Move from the top of the head and down the sides, to the neck, sides and forehead and up towards the top of the head. Remember to start brushing at the roots of the hair; the glands of your own scalp produce the best anti-dryness grooming oil available. By completing the strokes in one movement, oil is evenly distributed. However, if you have long hair, stroke only halfway, then hold the hair with one hand and complete the stroke with the other hand holding the brush. The problem with a continuous stroke on long hair is that of placing too much stress on the hair shaft and root, which can cause breakage.

The best type of brush to use is one made of natural bristle (usually boar). Just like your hair, the bristle is made of natural keratin, and will catch dirt and debris in the same way that your hair does. The dirt is absorbed by the bristles and removed from the hair. A nylon brush will not accomplish the same cleaning process. When the natural bristle brush gets dirty, just scrub it with a dry towel, or wipe the bristles with a towel after each brushing. Natural bristles have rounded ends, which is easier on the scalp and the hair shaft than the sharp bristles found on most nylon brushes. If you do purchase a nylon brush, make sure that the bristles have rounded ends. Natural bristle brushes are commonly available in natural foods stores, Chinese community stores and often in drugstores. Wooden combs, also available in health food stores and in Chinese stores, keep out static, which can be a problem for certain types of hair.

Conclusion

REMEMBER, halting and reversing hair loss is not an overnight affair. It may take months before improvements are noted, and could take a year before any new growth is apparent. In any case there are no guarantees. The key to success is daily hair care, a must for anyone with problem scalp or hair. A condition that took a lifetime to develop cannot be reversed in a matter of days or weeks. The techniques you choose to apply must be used consistently and rigorously. Haphazard, occasional therapy will have little or no effect.

In attempting to reverse hair loss it is wise to think in terms of synergy—the whole is greater than the sum of its parts. The more multi-layered your approach the greater your chances of success. Eliminating the causative factors under your control (e.g. smoking, excess salt consumption, excess cholesterol, high stress levels), combined with dietary changes, nutritional supplementation, scalp stimulation, externally applied formulas, and proper hair care and hygiene can accomplish far more than any isolated approach or technique. You are the experiment, and you are biochemically unique. Therefore a certain amount of trial and error is inevitable. To conclude we shall detail a basic routine designed to minimize hair loss, including both internal and external remedies. Of course, some personalization is necessary. Find the combination that works best for you and stick with it.

External

Follicle cleaning is critical to preventing fallage. While Polysorbate 80 has the best researched track record, it is somewhat awkward to apply. Jojoba Oil performs the same function of cleansing the follicles and is much easier to use, as it can be left on all night, doesn't stain, and washes out easily. It also regulates sebum production; preventing the scalp from becoming too dry or too oily, and revitalizes the hair shaft. Rosemary or peppermint oil may be added to the jojoba oil to stimulate circulation.

For a deeper cleaning action try alternating jojoba oil with apple cider vinegar. Apple cider vinegar should be rubbed into the scalp at full strength, and left on for fifteen minutes before shampooing. Cider vinegar normalizes the acid mantle on the scalp and kills off any bad bacteria that may be breeding in the buildup of dead skin cells.

Circulation: Bending over from the waist and gently brushing the entire scalp will enhance circulation and clean dead skin and debris which clogs the follicles from the scalp. If you have dead cell buildup on the scalp, flaking, and/or an itchy scalp it is important to shampoo regularly to aid in keeping the follicles unplugged.

Internal

Vegetal Silica: 500 mg, three per day
Saw Palmetto Berry Extract: Up to 160 mg Standardized Extract, twice per day
Vitamin A with Beta Carotene. (Specify natural source)
Vitamin C: At least 500 mg per day. (Specify 'Buffered')
Vitamin E. At least 400 iu per day (Specify 'Natural Source')
A multi-mineral complex, including Calcium and Magnesium, and Zinc.

Nothing so effectively prevents hair loss due to breakage as Vegetal Silica. Take Saw Palmetto Berry Extract for its proven ability to prevent the formation of DHT. The three vitamins (A, C, E) are the best researched and proven antioxidants. By scavenging the free radicals that cause cellular degeneration they naturally ward off cancer and heart disease, and also help prevent premature aging and the attendant hair loss. Vitamin C also supports the function of the adrenal glands, helping to combat the excess androgens produced by these glands when under stress. Calcium and Magnesium aid in stress prevention. Zinc helps to prevent the conversion of testosterone to DHT. All other major macro minerals should be represented along with trace minerals.

Essential Fatty Acids

Essential Fatty Acids are best taken in the form of Flax and Evening Primrose Oils. Alternate or take them together. Fish oils are another good source. Take supplements or eat fish at least twice per week. EFAs are found predominantly in the deep water fish including salmon, herring, mackerel, trout, or sardines. EFAs support immune functions, prevent premature aging, and regulate sebum functions, keeping the skin and hair healthy and vibrant. Because of the link between fats, EFAs, and the formation of DHT surrounding prostate problems and Male Pattern Baldness this is perhaps the most important area in which to exercise dietary controls. In order to raise and maintain adequate EFA levels one must also restrict the intake of 'bad' fats.

Join "The Hairnet"

YOU ARE INVITED TO JOIN 'THE HAIRNET', a quarterly newsletter containing the latest scientific information on hair loss prevention. These days new information on hair loss comes and goes in the blink of an eye. We'll help you sort out what works and what doesn't, and at the same time provide vital cultural and historical perspective.

We encourage dialogue. Members are invited to submit letters and questions, and we'll do our best to get you the most current and relevant information available.

Your first newsletter will include part one of 'The Oriental Approach to Hair Loss'. This article covers the ancient Zen Buddhist medicinal tradition of Japan, and offers their advice on the causes of and remedies for hair loss. Part two will cover the Chinese tradition, including acupuncture, herbs, and other prevention techniques.

Subscriptions are $14 US ($18 Cdn) per year, including postage. If we publish your letter or question you will receive one free copy.

Subscribe today!
Moss Rock Press
P.O. Box 35060
Hillside Postal Outlet
Victoria, BC
Canada   v8t 5G2

Bibliography*

Adams, Ruth, with Murray, Frank
Body, Mind, and B-Vitamins (Fourth Edition);
Los Angeles, Pinnacle Books, 1972.

Airola, Paavo, Stop Hair Loss (Twelfth Edition);
Phoenix, Health Plus Publishers, 1965.

Balch, James F, M.D., with Balch, Phyllis A.,
GNC Prescription for Nutritional Healing;
New York, Avery Publishing Group, 1990

Barolet, Randall, with Bensky, Dan,
Chinese Herbal Medicine Formulas; Seattle, Eastland Press, 1990

Berry, Neville, The World's Greatest Collection of Hair Loss Remedies;
Glan Publishing, 1990

Bragg, Paul C., with Bragg, Patricia,
Apple Cider Vinegar Health System,
Santa Barbara, Health Science, 1990

Calbom, Cherie, Juicing for Life;
New York, Avery Publishing Group, 1992

Chaitow, Leon, Prostate Troubles;
London, Thorson's Publishing Group, 1988

Chapman, J.B., M.D. and Perry, Edward L., M.D.
The Biochemical Handbook; St. Louis, Formur Publishing, 1976

Dunne, Lavon J., Nutrition Almanac (Third Edition);
New York, McGraw Hill, 1990

Hanssen, Maurice, The Healing Power of Pollen (Fourth Edition);
London, Thorson Pub., 1979

Heinerman, John, Aloe Vera, Jojoba, and Yuca;
Connecticut, Keats Publishing, 1982

Kaufman, Klaus, Silica, The Forgotten Nutrient;
Burnaby, BC, Alive Books, 1990

Khalsa, Siri, Nutrition News Volume Eight, Number Twelve;
Pomona, Ca., 1985

Kloss, Jethro, Back to Eden; New York, Benedict Lust Pub., 1971

Kushi, Michio, The Macrobiotic Way of Natural Healing;
Boston, East West Publications, 1978

Lee, William H. The Book of Raw Fruits and Vegetable Juices and
Drinks; Conneticut, Keats Publishing, 1982

Linde, Shirley, The Whole Health Catalogue (Third Edition);
Ottawa, McClelland and Stewart, 1977

Lucas, Richard, Nature's Medicines (Fourth Edition);
New York, Award Books, 1966

Lust, John B. The Herb Book (Thirteenth Edition);
New York, Bantam Books, 1980

——————Drink Your Troubles Away; New York, Benedict Lust Pub., 1967

Mindell, Earl, Vitamin Bible; New York, Warner Books, 1985

Morgan, Dr. Brian L., with Morgan, Roberta, Hormones;
Los Angeles, The Body Press, 1989

Pearson, Durk, with Shaw, Sandy, Life Extension;
   New York, Warner Books, 1982

Robbins, John, Diet for a New America;
   Walpole, New Hampshire, Stillpoint Pub., 1987

Rohlfing, Carla, "Thin, Thinner, Thinnest" Longevity, Volume One,
   Number Twelve, p.55-56, Sept., 1989

Segal, Darryl R., Hair For Life (Third Edition);
   Richmond, BC   Copyright by the Author, 1984

Stein, Irene, Royal Jelly; London, Thorson's Pub, 1989

Tenney, Louise, Today's Herbal Health (Second Edition);
   Utah, Woodland Books, 1983

Tierra, Michael, The Way of Herbs; Santa Cruz, Unity Press, 1980

Trattler, Dr. Ross, Better Health Through Natural Healing;
   New York, McGraw-Hill, 1985

Treben, Maria Health From God's Garden;
   Vermont, Healing Arts Press, 1985

Vogel, A, M.D. Swiss Nature Doctor (Forty Fourth Edition);
   Switzerland, 1952

Wade, Carlson, Magic Minerals; New York, Parker Publishing, 1967

————— Natural Hormones: The Secret of Youthful Health;
   New York, Parker Publishing, 1972

Weller, Stella, Super Healthy Hair, Skin, and Nails;
   London, Harper Collins, 1991

*For further information on these and other titles,
phone 1-604-325-2888 in the US or Canada.*

Up-date your knowledge of Fats & Healing with

Dr. Johanna Budwig

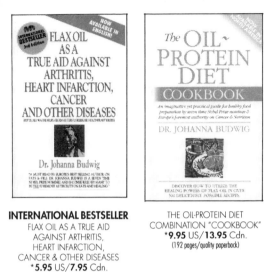

INTERNATIONAL BESTSELLER
FLAX OIL AS A TRUE AID
AGAINST ARTHRITIS,
HEART INFARCTION,
CANCER & OTHER DISEASES
*5.95 US/7.95 Cdn.
(64 pages/booklet)

THE OIL-PROTEIN DIET
COMBINATION "COOKBOOK"
*9.95 US/13.95 Cdn.
(192 pages/quality paperback)

Scientist, author & lecturer_ Dr. Budwig is <u>one of the foremost</u> authorities on Fat Metabolism.

Few people have had a greater impact on the medical community and modern nutritional science than this world-renowned pioneer and seven time Nobel Prize nominee.

- *Learn about "Good Fats & Bad Fats"*
- *Find out how fats govern all aspects of the human body.*
- *Discover the highly beneficial "Oil-Protein Diet"*
- *Read about Cancer Research and Fat Metabolism.*
- *Select nutritionally important foods.*
- *Learn the proper use of fats in daily cooking.*

Ask for these titles at your bookstore !

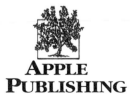

APPLE PUBLISHING

For further information phone:
1-604-325-2888 or fax **1-604-322-6978**

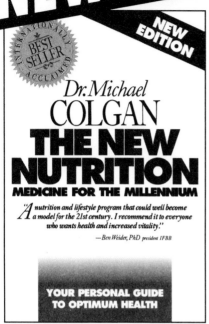